A Clinician's Companion

A Study Guide for Effective and Humane Patient Care

A Clinician's Companion

A Study Guide for Effective and Humane Patient Care

Joseph S. Alpert, M.D.
Professor of Medicine,
Department of Medicine,
University of Massachusetts
Medical School;
Director, Division of
Cardiovascular Medicine,
University of Massachusetts
Medical Center,
Worcester, Massachusetts

Stephen M. Wittenberg, M.D.
Associate Clinical
Professor of Medicine,
Tufts University School of Medicine,
Boston; Attending Cardiologist,
Baystate Medical Center,
Springfield, Massachusetts

Little, Brown and Company
Boston/Toronto

Library of Congress Catalog Card
No. 86-80820

ISBN 0-316-03511-4

Printed in the United States
of America

DON

To Sally, Alison, Andrew, Helle, Eva, and Niels

Contents

IV. Medical Ethics

Appendixes

Preface

In an era when physicians are often seen as adversaries rather than allies, it is important for them to reaffirm their traditional role as professionals who provide humane as well as expert health care. The technical advances in medicine in this half of the twentieth century have been astounding. Certainly, when patients are unhappy, they are not objecting to these advances. Patients also recognize that the cost of these advances is high and that honest attempts are being made to contain costs. Why then are patients discontented? If it is not the new knowledge or its high cost that has pushed physicians and patients apart, it must be the manner in which that knowledge is delivered to the bedside. It must be that we have sacrificed some of the art of medicine in our efforts to advance the science of medicine.

Physicians and patients must be brought closer together if patients are to be comfortable with their physicians and if physicians are to derive satisfaction from patient care. Neither benefit in an adversarial situation; both gain when a warm human relationship forms the matrix in which modern technology is used. In this book, we address some topics that can be gathered loosely under the heading "practical medical humanism." They represent the soft side of medical skill and, therefore, often tend to be taken less seriously or even ignored in medical textbooks. However, as essayist Norman Cousins has so aptly pointed out, it is ironic that the hard material of medical education quickly becomes obsolete, whereas this soft material remains ever useful and relevant.

If the tone of some of these chapters has too moralistic a ring for some readers, we apologize. The issues we address are, in fact, more important than the solutions we suggest. We recognize that other approaches are as valid as our own. Our primary goal is to stimulate increased concern and questioning by physicians about these issues and to underscore the need for understanding, compassion, and kindness in this technologic era. We would be pleased if this little book could serve as a core curriculum or study guide for courses in medical humanism. No matter how it is used, our hope is that it will contribute toward a humanizing trend in modern medicine and will thereby help to close the gap between physician and patient once again.

This book is directed primarily to young physicians—medical

students, house officers, and early practitioners—who are still in the process of acquiring their own style of medical practice. We hope that in some small way, this text will enable them to deliver high quality, compassionate care to their patients.

Many individuals aided us during the planning and writing of this book. We would like to acknowledge the constant intellectual and emotional support of our wives and the stimulating criticism of colleagues Roberta Berrien, M.D., Deborah Gilman, M.D., Lily Peng, Ira S. Ockene, M.D., John A. Paraskos, M.D., and James E. Dalen, M.D. Patient, accurate assistance with the manuscript was given by Marilyn Parks and James A. Krosschell.

J.S.A.
S.M.W.

A Clinician's Companion

A Study Guide for Effective and Humane Patient Care

I. Prerequisites for Clinicians

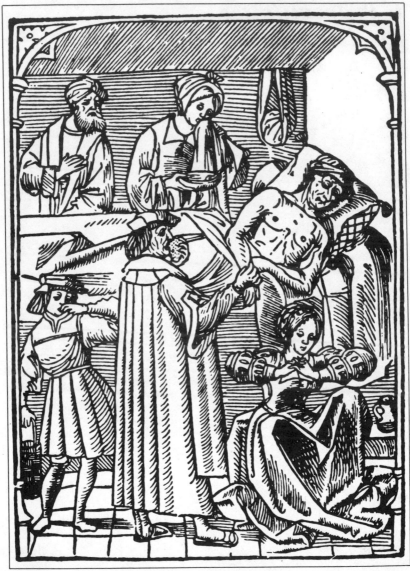

This German woodcut of the fifteenth century shows a physician
visiting a plague victim. Note that
the physician is taking the patient's
pulse (often the only part of the
modern physical examination that
was performed at that time). In addition, note that the physician
holds a sponge to his nose. This
was soaked in vinegar or perfume
and prevented the contagious
miasma, or vapor, from reaching
the physician's nose. Other
assistants or family members also
protect their noses. (From H. W.
Haggard. The Lame, the Halt, and
the Blind. *New York: Harper &
Brothers, 1932. P. 198.)*

1. Clinical Judgment and the Evaluation of Patients

It is widely believed that the work performed by scientists is totally objective, consisting of collection and examination of "facts" that reflect the real world. Traditional Newtonian physics courses teach students how to solve problems that have only one correct answer. For example, the student may be asked to calculate the velocity of an object of known mass at a known point in time after the object is dropped from an airplane. If the student employs the correct formula and performs the calculations correctly, the one "correct" answer will be obtained. Although this type of problem may be useful for teaching students the principles of mechanics, it also conveys a subtle message that may cause difficulties if the student goes on to study clinical medicine (i. e., objective data are usually available, and given these data, one correct answer is possible).

The development of quantum physics in the twentieth century has led to a reexamination of the manner in which the so-called facts of science are viewed. German nuclear physicist Werner Heisenberg (1901–) has written extensively on uncertainty in modern physics. Heisenberg points out that it is impossible to determine at one moment in time both the position and the velocity of an electron spinning around an atomic nucleus. Heisenberg demonstrated that the energy focused on the electron in order to observe it altered the velocity or the position of this atomic particle. This is referred to as the Heisenberg uncertainty principle. Of course, one can make a probability statement concerning the *likely* position and velocity of the electron. There is, however, a definite chance that the experimenting scientist's statement concerning the electron's position and velocity is wrong.

The Heisenberg uncertainty principle can be applied in a variety of scientific arenas including medical science. Its message is clear: The scientist *alters* the *milieu by his or her very presence.* This occurs in several ways. First, the observations of any particular physician are subjective. They are rooted in genetic characteristics, past experiences, current situations. They are influenced by the attitudes of family, friends, and colleagues. Next, they are limited by the appropriateness of that physician's observational tools. Finally, the actions taken on the basis of the observations derive from subjective judgments, and these actions themselves affect the illness or experiment—in a manner similar to that illustrated by Heisenberg for observed electrons. Thus, the physician must accept the concept that alleged facts, perceived as existing in the "real" world, have probably been altered to some degree by the very act of observation. These alleged facts are not totally objective and do not exist without reference to the observer.

Since physicians approach data from a point of view and since they change it in the very act of approaching it, we can readily understand why the history of medicine is filled with examples of theories and therapies that enjoyed brief or prolonged popularity only to fade and be forgotten. Much of what we consider fact will no doubt suffer the same fate. Thus, clinicians need to remind themselves constantly of the evanescent nature of many medical theories and therapies and of the tentative nature of their ideas in any particular case. The implication is that *physicians should embrace new therapies only after great scrutiny and should similarly make a specific diagnosis or prescribe a therapy open-mindedly, realizing that changes may have to be made.*

Does this mean that the physician works in a shifting world of kaleidoscopic dimensions with no real facts and with subjectivity everywhere? In fact, the situation is not as frightening as it may sound at first. More objective methods of decision making are being developed through research on decision analysis (Pauker, 1980). In the meantime, medical knowledge, experience, and common sense can assist the clinician in deciding on *the most probable diagnosis* and in formulating a strategy to confirm or refute it. These attributes can also guide the physician in constructing a treatment plan that will *probably* be effective. It is, however, important to keep the word *probable* in mind at all times and to realize that anything that one does may change the natural history of the illness. An example follows:

A 28-year-old graduate student comes to the hospital emergency room complaining of pleuritic chest pain, fever, and chills. A third-year medical student is the first person to interrogate and examine the patient. The medical student has limited experience and fears that the patient has a serious condition. Extensive diagnostic tests (complete blood count, automated blood chemistry panel, blood cultures, chest x ray, and ventilation-perfusion scan of the lung) are ordered. Before all these tests can be performed, a senior resident reviews the case with the medical student. The resident obtains a more focused history from the patient. It is learned that two other family members had similar but transient symptoms. Moreover, the resident tells the medical student that this is the sixth patient seen that day in the emergency room with the same symptoms. In addition, other patients with a similar transient illness have been seen in the emergency room during the last week. The resident concludes from her experience and the patient's history that this individual has a viral illness that is perhaps influenza. She chooses the two tests that are most likely to support her diagnosis and at the same time screen for a more serious problem (i.e., a complete blood count and a chest x ray). She cancels the other tests. When the tests return negative, the resident allows the patient to return home with only symptomatic treatment.

The combination of knowledge, experience, and common sense enables the resident to recognize a probable viral illness passing through the patient's family and community. Of course, the experienced physician is aware of the uncertainty involved in making the diagnosis of viral syndrome in this patient. There is a small but definite probability that this patient does not have influenza but rather a serious bacterial infection or a pulmonary embolus. In sending the patient home rather than admitting him or her to the hospital, the resident is intruding into the illness, whatever it is. Even in the act of reassuring the patient that this illness is in all likelihood a viral illness that will soon disappear, the resident emphasizes that the patient should return to the emergency room for further evaluation if the symptoms increase in severity or fail to abate over the next 2 to 3 days. The resident realizes that she cannot determine the cause of the patient's illness with total accuracy. Rather, a probable diagnosis is made, and symptomatic therapy is prescribed for the patient; at the same time, a policy is instituted that should lead the patient to return for further evaluation if the illness fails to follow the usual course of a viral syndrome.

Decisions made in an environment fraught with uncertainty should never be considered as objective and incontrovertible facts. Rather, such decisions should be viewed as *probability statements* (i.e., the favored horse *will probably* win the race). New information or further examination of existing data may lead to an alteration in the probability statement. This case presentation also illustrates two opposite but complementary principles of good clinical judgment: (1) *The physician should not multiply causes, tests, or treatments without good reason, and (2) the physician should not rest the case without reluctance, but should rather continue the debate.*

Another aspect of clinical judgment relates to the manner in which the physician approaches the patient. Biased, intellectually arrogant, or unfeeling attitudes on the part of the physician represent an error in clinical judgment since such attitudes interfere with data collection and appropriate therapy. Consider the following example:

A fatigued emergency room physician is called to see a semiconscious patient with a history of chronic alcohol abuse. The physician smells alcohol on the patient's breath and performs a cursory examination. He tells the family, "This man is just drunk. Take him home and let him sleep it off." The family sheepishly complies and, in their embarrassment, forgets to tell the physician that the patient had complained of inability to use his right leg for several hours before he was found in his bedroom in a semiconscious state. The next morning, the patient is brought to the emergency room deeply comatose. Subsequent evaluation reveals that the patient has suffered a major cerebral hemorrhage.

The emergency room physician exercised poor clinical judgment in evaluating and treating this patient. The physician became annoyed and jumped to the conclusion that the patient's state of consciousness was due to alcohol ingestion alone. The annoyed physician failed to obtain a piece of historical information that might have led to the correct diagnosis. The *physician's clinical judgment was impaired by personal feelings about chronic alcoholism.*

Clinical judgment usually requires medical knowledge, some experience, common sense, and an awareness of one's own biases. It may also require moral reasoning. Consider the following situation:

A 40-year-old woman with 3 children comes to the emergency room with a 6-hour history of abdominal pain and nausea. Examination reveals a temperature of 100°F and rebound tenderness of the abdomen in the right lower quadrant. The urinalysis is negative; the white blood count is elevated to 14,000 with a shift to the left. The patient's only previous operation was a tonsillectomy as a child. A tentative diagnosis of acute appendicitis is made, and a surgeon is called for further evaluation. The surgeon concurs and advises immediate operation. The patient requests a tubal ligation if she is to undergo surgery. The surgeon, for religious reasons, feels that he cannot comply. Obviously, the surgeon can proceed from here in more than one way. He can simply state that he cannot do the tubal ligation. He can, on the other hand, suggest that the patient call in someone else who can do both procedures at the same time.

This particular moral dilemma is fairly simple. Other more complicated issues arise frequently. An example is a patient with venereal disease contracted from someone other than the patient's spouse. The patient may have had sexual intercourse with the spouse since contracting the illness, yet may request that the physician not inform the spouse. This situation presents medical and moral challenges. Sheehan and his colleagues have been studying determinants of good physician performance. They have found that a highly developed capacity for moral reasoning correlates more strongly with physician performance than do examinations of factual knowledge (Sheehan, 1980).

Working Up the Patient

The process by which physicians determine the pathologic entity from which the patient suffers is often referred to as the work-up. History, physical examination, and laboratory tests are all used by the physician during the work-up to arrive at a probable diagnosis of the patient's problem. Thereafter, therapeutic measures are instituted. Ideally, therapy should be based on an understanding of the pathophysiologic process occurring within the patient. Medical or surgical therapy attempts to reverse, at least in part, this pathophysiologic process. All patients should receive a thoughtful work-up. In some individuals, the work-up is short, while in others, the process is more lengthy. The process can be best understood by examining some examples.

A previously healthy and athletic 15-year-old student who fell on her arm while playing basketball complains of severe tenderness on the dorsal aspect of the left wrist and is reluctant to move the fingers of the left hand because of pain. There is considerable tenderness over the distal head of the left radius. An x ray of the left wrist reveals a nondisplaced fracture of the distal head of the radius.

In this patient, the work-up was quite short. This patient was a healthy teenager who suffered simple trauma to the left wrist and sustained an uncomplicated fracture of the left radius. A complete history and physical examination were not required. Rather, the history and physical examination were both focused on the traumatic event that occurred. The selected laboratory evaluation is also quite simple: a radiographic evaluation of the bones of the left wrist. A more extensive work-up is not indicated in this patient.

A 50-year-old man seeks medical advice because of recurring episodes of nagging chest discomfort. His best friend has recently died from a myocardial infarction. The chest discomfort is substernal, occurs with episodes of exertion or emotional turmoil, and lasts 5 to 10 minutes. The discomfort is described as "burning, like indigestion." The patient has smoked two packs of cigarettes daily for 20 years. He has not seen a physician for 10 years. The physical examination is unremarkable. Supporting laboratory work includes a normal resting electrocardiogram and chest x ray, a serum cholesterol of 290 mg per dl, and a markedly abnormal, or positive, electrocardiographic exercise test. The patient's diagnosis following this work-up is angina pectoris, probably secondary to arteriosclerotic coronary artery disease.

As is usually the case, the diagnosis is already evident with a reasonably high degree of certainty after the patient's history has been obtained. The physical examination is often normal in patients with this condition; laboratory data (the exercise test) confirms the presence of myocardial ischemia during exercise. The elevated serum cholesterol and the history of smoking are factors that are felt to be involved in the etiology of this disease process, and most physicians try to eliminate such risk factors for coronary artery disease from their healthy patients as well as from individuals in whom clinically evident sequelae of arteriosclerosis are already present. The chest x ray was obtained to see if the heart was enlarged and if there was any evidence of heart failure. In contrast to the first example, this work-up consisted of a detailed history, a complete physical examination, and a number of laboratory tests. This work-up should be contrasted with that of the next patient.

A 50-year-old man who drinks and smokes heavily complains of dyspnea on effort. On examination, he is noted to have distended neck veins, basilar rales, an S3 gallop, and peripheral edema. The diagnostic possibilities causing these signs and symptoms include congestive cardiomyopathy secondary to chronic alcohol abuse (likely), chronic obstructive pulmonary disease with cor pulmonale (likely), and pulmonary embolism (less likely). Other diagnostic entities are considerably less likely (e.g., left atrial myxoma and constrictive pericarditis). The work-up of this patient begins with noninvasive tests (e.g., chest x ray, echocardiography, or nuclear study of left ventricular function and pulmonary function studies, which are harmless and less costly than invasive tests (e.g., cardiac catheterization). If the noninvasive tests do not demonstrate the sought-for condition, the more risky and expensive tests are ordered as the search continues for the patient's diagnosis.

This patient is not as straightforward as the first two examples, since he may have *all three* of our most likely diagnostic conditions simultaneously. His work-up might eventually involve both noninvasive and invasive testing. In general, the more straightforward and simple the work-up, the better. *Simple is good.* Thus, the simplest test likely to give an answer should be ordered first. The more complex the work-up, the greater the chance for confusion secondary to false-positive laboratory results. Each of the first two patients described had a single disease process, enabling the physician to keep the work-up simple. Obviously, some patients have multiple diseases or an obscure condition; either of these situations leads to much more complex and lengthy work-ups, as in the third patient example.

One can minimize complexity and maximize effectiveness by following two other precepts: (1) *Common things occur commonly,* and (2) *serious treatable conditions must not be missed.* In planning and organizing the testing process, the physician constructs a list of diagnostic possibilities known as the differential diagnosis. Using the rules Simple is good, Common things occur commonly, and Serious treatable conditions must not be missed, laboratory tests are chosen in such a fashion as to confirm or exclude the most likely and important diseases first.

How does the physician rank his or her diagnostic possibilities? Usually he or she will begin by considering as most likely those things that occur most often in the patient's overall life-setting and are most important not to overlook. For example, chest pain in middle-aged men must raise the consideration of coronary artery disease, but chest pain in a healthy young person is often due to some pleuritic or pericarditic process. Next, specific conditions present in characteristic ways. For example, the chest discomfort of myocardial infarction usually begins in the center of the chest in the region of the sternum. The discomfort often radiates to the neck, jaw, and inner aspects of the left or both arms. The patient often feels nauseated and breaks out in a cold sweat. Chills and fever do not occur. Pneumonia, on the other hand, produces chest pain that is usually localized to one side of the chest, often in the back of the chest. The chest discomfort associated with pneumonia is the result of pleuritic irritation and is, therefore, made worse by deep inspiration. The knowledgeable physician seeks information from the patient in order to define the characteristics of the chest pain.

In summary, the physician constructs a ranked list of diagnostic possibilities for each patient based on the ailment that seems to fit the symptom complex that the patient manifests best, the overall life-setting in which the illness occurs, and the importance of not overlooking a serious, remediable condition.

Cost-Benefit and the Differential Diagnosis

Another factor that should be considered in the work-up of a patient's presenting complaint is the ratio of cost to benefit. Cost in this context refers both to economic cost and to pain and suffering. Both entities extract something from the patient: money or physical or psychologic distress. *The physician needs to know the potential economic or personal cost of a particular diagnostic test and the likelihood that the test will be definitive in making the diagnosis or changing the treatment.* Ideally, an inexpensive and painless test is best; however, the test chosen will depend on risk-benefit as well as cost and discomfort.

The physician should consider whether the results of a given test will alter the patient's therapy or comfort. No test that is not associated with a reasonable likelihood of altering either therapy or patient comfort should be performed on a patient. It should be stressed that patient comfort has both physical and psychologic or emotional components. Therefore, a test that does not alter therapy, but that confirms a rather benign diagnostic entity and eliminates a frightening one is certainly worth performing. Two examples elucidate this reasoning:

A 35-year-old, high-strung man complains of intermittent episodes of constipation and diarrhea. After close questioning, the physician feels that the patient has benign irritable colon. However, a distant cousin has died of complications of ulcerative colitis, and the patient is very fearful that he has this condition. The physician performs a colonoscopic examination and obtains biopsies of several areas of colonic mucosa that appear inflamed. The colonoscopic examination and the biopsy results are negative for ulcerative colitis. The benefit of the colonoscopic examination outweighs the risk and the economic and personal cost.

A 75-year-old woman is found to have metastatic ovarian cancer. She deteriorates despite aggressive therapy over 10 months and becomes essentially bedridden and semicomatose. Intermittent episodes of diarrhea and constipation develop, but colonoscopy is not considered indicated by her physician because it will not change the therapeutic program, which is essentially supportive at this time. The expense and discomfort associated with colonoscopy are not felt to be indicated in this terminally ill patient. Cost (economic and personal) outweighs benefit.

Another rule is *It is foolish and wasteful to order two tests that produce the same information.* If the physician has obtained an echocardiogram, which allows accurate evaluation of ventricular function in a patient with heart disease, a radionuclide ventriculogram is not needed since the latter test yields information similar to that derived from the echocardiogram. The two tests are (in this instance but not always) redundant. The rational work-up is like a carefully reasoned argument in a debate: It proceeds logically from one point to the next without redundancy or confusion.

The Conclusion
of the Work-Up

Every diagnostic work-up should conclude with a *thoughtful* review of the data and the conclusions drawn from the information obtained. Frequently, this thoughtful review is an ongoing process occurring throughout the work-up. Nevertheless, a summary of the work-up placed in the patient's chart is invaluable to future physicians who will deal with this patient. Inpatients always have such a summary, the discharge summary, which is dictated when the patient is discharged from the hospital. Outpatients who undergo an extensive diagnostic work-up should likewise have a brief summary of the information obtained and the conclusions drawn from the diagnostic evaluation. Finally, it should be emphasized that not all diagnostic work-ups lead to firm conclusions. The physician may still be puzzled, and the diagnosis may still be unclear even after a careful and rational diagnostic evaluation. In this setting, it is often useful to discuss the patient with a colleague. Many times, the ensuing discussion produces new insights that lead to a resolution of the diagnostic enigma. Often, the physician who has been wrestling with the diagnostic problem will see a solution to the dilemma during the presentation of the patient to a colleague. Many group practices and hospitals institutionalize such discussions in the form of conferences (e. g., clinical-pathologic or morbidity and mortality rounds). Such discussions usually lead to an increase in physician experience and hence to improved patient care.

Suggested Reading

Bursztajn, H., Feinbloom, R. I., Hamm, R. M., and Brodsky, A. *Medical Choices, Medical Chances—How Patients, Families and Physicians Can Cope With Uncertainty.* New York: Delacorte, 1981. Pp. 20–84.
Feinstein, A. R. *Clinical Judgment.* Huntington, N. Y.: Kreiger, 1967. Pp. 21–30, 291–305.
Judge, R. D., Zuidema, G. D., and Fitzgerald, F. T. *Clinical Diagnosis: A Physiologic Approach.* Boston: Little, Brown, 1982. Chaps. 1,2,21,22.
Pauker, S. G., and Kassirer, J. P. The threshold approach to clinical decision making. *N. Engl. J. Med.* 302:1109, 1980.
Pellegrino, E. D., and Thomasma, D. C. *A Philosophical Basis of Medical Practice,* New York: Oxford, 1981. Chap. 6.
Sheehan, T. J., Husted, S., Candee, D., Cook, C., and Bargen, M. Moral judgment as a predictor of clinical performance. *Eval. Health Professions* 3:393, 1980.

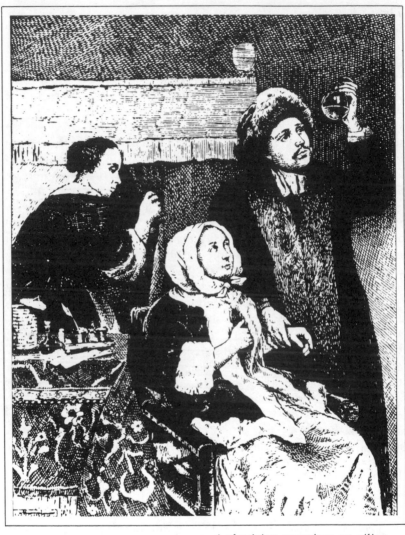

A physician examines an ailing woman. The diagnostic evaluation consists of taking the pulse and examining a sample of the patient's urine. (By Gaspard Netscher, 1639–1684.)

2. Clinical Care

The patient is neither a disease to be discussed nor a showcase of pathologic interest, nor a dispassionate bystander. He is a sick person in the
alien environment of the hospital, disturbed by his illness and involved
in it at least as much as the doctors. He is anxious to know what is happening, entitled to find out, and generally able to make helpful contribu-
tions to all aspects of his clinical management. . . . the failure to give
adequate concern to the patient is detrimental to the art of medical
education and of patient care.

Alvan R. Feinstein
Clinical Judgment

Medicine has been called a service profession, since the physician
serves the patient. The word "serve" implies subservience. This is
misleading and masks the great power of the servant over the
served. A similar situation prevails in other service professions such
as government and education. Take, for example, the often used
phrase of presidents: "It is my honor to serve the people." This
pronouncement makes more palatable, but only thinly veils, the
great power of that office.

The power of the physician rests in her or his role as guardian of
health and warrior against illness. Medicine is truly a service profession only if the physician continually strives to use this power in the
best interest of the patient. Schools of medicine and hospital training programs have long emphasized the importance of accurate and
current medical knowledge in this endeavor. They have paid less attention to the manner in which physicians use their knowledge and
skill. This has been termed the *art* of medicine, somehow implying
that it is a luxury, not a necessity. Yet, it is the manner of delivery of
clinical care that most often determines a patient's level of comfort,
degree of confidence, and willingness to cooperate and, not infrequently, the medical outcome itself. This chapter addresses some
aspects of the art of clinical care.

Bedside Manner
Bedside manner is a term used much more frequently in the first
half of this century than the second half. This is because, in the past,
bedside manner was all the physician had to offer in many illnesses.
In the current high-technology era, more tangible treatment is available, and one rarely hears about bedside manner. However, there

are some things the physician can do to make his or her visit to the bedside more respectful and more pleasant for the patient. Examples include knocking on the door if it is shut, pulling the curtain or closing the door before beginning an examination, giving a patient time if she or he is in the bathroom at that moment, and apologizing if the visit is at mealtime. All of us can think of other courtesies. In addition, it is nice to sit down on the bed or in a chair, rather than stand at the foot of the bed. It has been shown that patients report more time spent by a physician when she or he sits down, even if the actual time is the same. It is important to greet the patient, perhaps exchange some small talk, and then try to elicit the patient's concerns before proceeding to one's own. Good bedside manner follows if the physician remembers that he or she is *visiting a person who is sick in bed,* not just seeing a patient.

Kindness and Respect

The physician-patient relationship is fraught with risk for the patient. The physician is in a position to declare sickness or wellness. She or he is also likely to prescribe discomfort or proscribe enjoyment. The patient, aware of these dangers, often faces the physician with a general sense of anxiety, some specific fears, a general type of hostility directed at the physician role, and a pledged resistance to possible unpleasant recommendations. Any one, let alone all, of these attitudes, can complicate the physician's goal of helping to maintain or restore the patient's health. A combination of kindness and respect is helpful in defusing anxiety, allaying fear, converting hostility into trust, and promoting cooperation. An example follows:

A 64-year-old woman seeks medical advice because of a 1-month history of blurred vision, thirst, and frequent urination. The patient is obese, but has felt well until recently. She has not seen a physician in many years. In fact, she would not have sought medical attention at all if her husband had not become annoyed and told her to "stop complaining about her symptoms and see a doctor." After arriving in the physician's waiting room, she encounters a 40-minute delay. Finally, a medical assistant comes to the window and beckons her toward an examining room. The medical assistant hands her a paper gown and says, "Take everything off from the waist up, and put this gown on." Once in the examining room, the patient becomes increasingly uncomfortable. She does not like disrobing because her obesity embarrasses her. She fears something serious, such as a brain tumor. She hates physicians anyway and always has. She will not let them "cut her up." She is perspiring profusely. The physician enters the room, introduces himself, and apologizes for his lateness. He shakes her hand and sits down at his desk. He notices the patient's perspiration and says, "It's very warm in here. Would you like me to turn down the heat?" She thanks him, but declines. The physician says, "Would you like to tell me how I can help you?" The patient begins to relax.

After taking a history, the physician says, "I would like to examine you," and beckons her toward the examining table. The patient comments that she will not be able to get up very gracefully because of her weight. The physician says, "Let me help you—the companies that make these tables must test them on Olympic athletes, not ordinary people. I'd like to see some of the designers get up on them gracefully." The patient smiles.

In this case report, the patient did not really want to see a physician. She was pushed into it and arrived feeling anxious, angry, and vulnerable. As is so often the case, the physician prolonged the patient's anxiety with his lateness. The patient approached the visit ashamed of her obesity and afraid of ridicule. The instructions to disrobe from the waist up and wait in a barely adequate paper gown eroded her remaining dignity. The physician began the visit by apologizing for his lateness, trying to demonstrate that he would treat her with dignity, making her aware of his sensitivity to her needs, and suggesting that he was there to help, not just to diagnose and treat. In other words, he approached her with kindness and respect rather than cool professionalism.

Many of these problems occur daily in physicians' offices. Every effort should be made to minimize them. This is best done by trying to put oneself in the patient's place (i.e., by developing empathy for the patient).

Empathy

Empathy implies the ability to put oneself into the other person's shoes—to feel as well as to grasp intellectually the other person's plight. Empathy should go beyond particular physican-patient encounters to the general role of patient. No one would go to a physician were it not for illness or fear of illness. This immediately places the patient in a dependent role with respect to the physician. The patient's uneasiness about the role and the situation is present by definition. Physician empathy for the patient role should also be there by definition. As the physician explores the patient's health status, it is important to get a feeling for the situation (i.e., to ascertain the emotional as well as the intellectual meaning to the patient of symptoms and signs). Possible treatment plans must be weighed in light of their feasibility for the patient as well as for the physician. During the encounter, the physician should try to change her or his image from one of healer to one of helper, thereby converting an atmosphere of rank and order to one of teamwork. Once a patient senses empathy from the physician, the patient's fears diminish since she or he knows the physician will act to minimize suffering. The following case illustrates medical competence without adequate empathy:

A 70-year-old woman from a small city seeks medical help for the recent onset of visual disturbances. The patient is sent for a computed tomography (CT) scan of the head at her local hospital. The CT scan shows a small, smooth-walled, probably benign mass not too far from the optic chiasm. The patient is told of this and advised to see a neurosurgeon. She is given several names, one in the small city where she lives and two in a neighboring larger city. She asks, "Which one would you choose, doctor?" She is told, "They are all excellent." She leaves the physician's office shaken by the news and worried about which consultant she should select. She feels helpless and does not quite know to whom to turn. Finally it occurs to her that she has a physician relative in a nearby city. She calls this physician and obtains a referral to a reputedly excellent neurologist at a major university hospital 2 hours away. She sees this neurologist, likes her, but is disappointed to find that the CT scan has to be repeated at the large medical center. The neurologist promises to call the patient as soon as she has the results. The patient and her husband stay at home, close to the telephone, for days. They are literally afraid to go out and miss the neurologist's call. As time passes, they become increasingly anxious and short-tempered. Intermittently, one or the other fights back tears of fear and anger. In fact, the neurologist has the results of the CT scan and knows that they support the original diagnosis of a benign lesion that is probably incidental rather than responsible for the symptoms and that can be safely watched rather than removed. However, the neurologist is very busy, and the call is delayed day after day.

In this report, the local physician and the neurologist were well meaning and competent. However, they failed to put themselves in the patient's place. The local physician should have responded to the patient's plea to designate a specific consultant. It is generally easier for a physician to identify the best person for the consultation than for a patient to do so. Subsequently, the neurologist should have kept her promise to call promptly. This could have averted a great deal of agony for the patient and her husband. The physician has many sick patients to worry about. This makes it difficult, but no less important, to remember that for any one patient, the problem is all consuming.

It is often in the setting of a prolonged problem where no medical solution is available that the physician's empathy is most sought and yet most difficult to give. An example follows:

A vigorous 75-year-old man undergoes emergency coronary bypass surgery for unstable angina and a high-grade left main coronary artery stenosis.

He is doing well from the cardiac standpoint, but does not come out of a coma postoperatively. In addition, his renal function deteriorates. The neurologic consultant, on the basis of the examination and the electroencephalogram (EEG), feels the coma is metabolic. Therefore, renal dialysis is begun, and gas exchange and fluid and electrolyte balance are carefully maintained. Days drag into weeks, but the patient remains in coma. The neurologist comes by and gives the patient a less than 3 percent chance of waking up. The family members, who maintain hope, are not ready to give up. They begin to grasp at straws. They say things like, "He opened his eyes." "He moved his legs." The family tries to call the neurologist but cannot reach him. They are referred by his office to the cardiologist. The cardiologist, when first contacted, says the neurologist would be better able to answer questions about the coma. The family again tries to contact the neurologist, but is told, "It is not good for too many doctors to deal with the family. The neurologist's note is in the chart." The cardiologist finally realizes that she will have to deal with the family. She begins to discuss code status and withdrawal of dialysis with the family. The family asks for another EEG. They ask numerous questions. Each day, they seek out the cardiologist with a look of hope. The cardiologist begins to dread the meetings. They always seem to make her late. They never seem to go anywhere. One day, the family speaks of the patient's previous vigor, of his wish not to be disabled, of his kindness to his family, of many things. The cardiologist listens and begins to understand the ordeal of the family in trying to let go. That day the family thanks the cardiologist for her kindness. Discussions continue, and several days later, the family requests that there be no resuscitation and that dialysis be stopped.

It is easy to rejoice with a patient who is recovering from an illness. It is much more difficult to remain faithful to a patient who is not getting well. The frustration of an impasse, the disillusionment of failure, and the indictment accompanying unmet expectations all tend to cause avoidance on the part of the physician. It is easier to be unavailable, or brief, or cool, than to face frustration. Yet if the victories are the physician's, so are the defeats. Empathetic practice is difficult when one is overcommitted and harassed. A great deal of suffering can be caused by placing this human aspect of practice lower in priority than some of the technical aspects. Conversely, a great deal of good can be done by giving patients and families time and concern and by showing empathy. Often, this involves only listening.

Listening

Listening skills are important in several different but related ways. Listening is essential in making the correct diagnosis. Listening may be even more important in helping the physician appreciate the meaning of the symptoms or illness to the patient. At times, just being listened to can be therapeutic for the patient. Finally, the listening process may convert a routine or even unpleasant patient into an interesting or appealing one. Cases are presented to illustrate these points.

LISTENING FOR DIAGNOSIS

Every physician knows the importance of the history in the evaluation of a patient. Every experienced physician also knows the difficulty in listening to everything the patient has to say. Yet it is often a word, a phrase, an unexpected comment, or a seemingly contradictory statement that helps the physician make the correct diagnosis when a common illness presents in an uncommon way or when an unusual illness is present. An example follows:

A 48-year-old man who lives in a small town seeks medical advice because of shortness of breath on effort. Physical examination reveals a blood pressure of 160/100 mm Hg, a grade II/VI systolic ejection murmur localized to the left sternal border, and an S4 gallop. Carotid pulsations are brisk. The electrocardiogram (ECG) is suggestive of left ventricular hypertrophy, and the chest x ray shows mild cardiomegaly. Since it is a small town, sophisticated diagnostic equipment is not available. The physician makes the diagnosis of hypertension and mild congestive heart failure. She begins the patient on a diuretic for blood pressure control and for treatment of the congestive heart failure. The patient calls a few days later and reports that the shortness of breath is worse. The physician then digitalizes the patient. Once again, the patient calls to report further aggravation of the shortness of breath. The physician obtains a chest x ray, which shows no evidence of pulmonary congestion. She becomes frustrated and begins to wonder if some of the patient's symptomatology is out of proportion to the illness (i.e., psychogenic). She tells the patient to give the therapy more time. The patient, in turn, is frustrated and frightened and seeks a consultant in a larger, neighboring city. The consultant makes the diagnosis of hypertrophic cardiomyopathy, thus explaining the contradictory symptoms.

This patient had an unusual, rather than a common, illness. His physician had undoubtedly seen very few patients like him. In addition, the special equipment needed to confirm the diagnosis was not readily at hand. However, had the physician seriously listened to the patient, she might have been prompted to look up conditions worsened by diuretics or digitalis or to seek help from a cardiologist colleague. The hypertrophic cardiomyopathy would have emerged quickly as a diagnostic possibility.

LISTENING TO DETERMINE
THE REASON FOR A VISIT
Not infrequently, a patient's fear of illness may be more the problem than the illness itself. In these cases, the patient presents with physical complaints but the physician finds no serious organic problem. The patient may be reticent to voice the fear or may not completely realize the fear. Careful listening may help the physician unearth the real problem. An example follows:

A 60-year-old man who underwent aortic valve replacement several years ago now presents with left upper chest and left arm pain. The pain is aggravated on movement of the extremity and is unrelated to other types of physical exertion. Cardiac examination is unremarkable, but there is some local tenderness in the left upper pectoral area. The physician assures the patient that the problem is not cardiac, but instead musculoskeletal. The patient concurs and admits that he has been required to lift heavier objects lately at work. Despite the reassurance, the patient is still tense and prolongs the visit with several extraneous matters. During the discussion, he casually asks the physician whether replaced heart valves ever burst. The physician pursues this and soon realizes that the patient is not really worried about the left chest pain per se but instead is concerned that heavy lifting will eventually cause the prosthetic heart valve to break. Specific reassurance that this never happens calms the patient.

If the physician had cut the patient off abruptly after it was clear that the problem was not serious, he or she might have missed the patient's real concern. Only continued listening revealed the patient's specific fear. Patients' reasons for visiting physicians have been divided by some people into the *ostensible reason for coming* and the *actual reason for coming*. This patient's ostensible reason for coming was chest pain, but the actual reason for coming was fear that his prosthetic aortic valve would burst.

LISTENING AS THERAPY
Sometimes listening, followed by a few understanding words, can be all the therapy that is necessary. Most people, including physicians, know this instinctively. However, physicians all too often trade their ordinary human instincts for technical skills. The following case illustrates how diagnostic skill coupled with empathetic listening can be highly therapeutic.

A 58-year-old woman arrives in the emergency room at 2 A.M. gasping for breath. The emergency room physician examines her and can find no abnormalities. Her lips and nails are pink, her lungs clear, her heart rate slightly increased but without significant murmurs or gallops. A chest x ray is un-remarkable, and blood studies including arterial blood gases are suggestive only of hyperventilation. The physician gently tells the patient that she can find no serious abnormality and asks her if anything has upset her. At this point, tears well up in her eyes, and she begins to sob. After a few minutes, she relates her story. "I have been married for 19 years and have two teen-age children. I am very fond of my family and have never wanted to hurt them. About 12 years ago, I met a man and fell in love with him. We have met secretly 2 or 3 times a year, and neither of us has told anyone for fear of destroying our families. A few days ago, I heard coincidentally that this man had died suddenly. I was devastated, but there was no one I could tell. I tried to appear normal to all around me. Tonight after going to bed, my heart began to race, and I became increasingly short of breath and was brought here. I don't know what to do, doctor. I am so sad." The emergen-cy room physician sits with her for a while and tells her she can understand what a great sense of loss she must feel. She allows her to talk and cry. When she leaves, her breathing is easy, and she seems much calmer. The physician gives her the name of someone to call for psychologic help.

In medical terminology, this woman's diagnosis was hyperventi-lation. Some people might have called her symptoms hysterical. Some physicians might have given her a bag to breathe into or a tranquilizer. In fact, what this patient needed more than anything else was someone to listen to her with empathy, kindness, and re-spect. Listening, in this example, was a very powerful therapeutic tool.

Listening and Empathy

At times, listening may be instrumental in helping the physician de-velop empathy for a seemingly unpleasant patient. We believe that the more a physician knows about a patient's suffering, the more likely the physician is to feel positively about the patient and, con-sequently, to have empathy for the patient. An example follows:

A 63-year-old man with a known seizure disorder controlled on medication is hospitalized with an uncomplicated myocardial infarction. His internist calls in a cardiologist and asks the cardiologist to take over the patient's care completely. The internist says he and the patient have never gotten along well, and this seems like an appropriate time to make a smooth transition. The cardiologist feels a bit trapped, but agrees to do it as a favor, soon realizing why the internist does not like the patient. He is unctuous and sar-castic. He often accompanies his statements with a nervous, annoying laugh. One day, the patient says something odd. He alludes to the fact that his boss often vents pent-up anger on him. The cardiologist listens as the patient tells about his role as whipping boy for a boss who does not have the nerve to speak up to his superiors at work. After the patient has rambled on a while, he suddenly stops and apologizes for spilling out his personal problems. "I cause everyone so much trouble with my seizures and now my heart." The cardiologist, who has become absorbed in the story, realizes that this man leads a miserable existence. He sees him as someone who feels he is worthless, and therefore, never dreams of confronting his boss's abuses. More importantly, instead of an unpleasant person, he sees before him a sad and suffering human being. He has an entirely different feeling for him.

This case illustrates the fact that empathy is not always automatic. Some people are not readily likable. Physicians concerned with medical or surgical problems need to learn what most psychiatrists already know. Listening often gives one enough insight to cut through unpleasant, superficial personality traits and see a patient's suffering. Many things in medicine, including listening, require compulsiveness and flexibility.

Compulsiveness
and Flexibility

Good clinical care requires a balance between compulsiveness and flexibility. Compulsiveness is emphasized in medical training, but the reasoning behind it is rarely discussed. There are some valid reasons for stressing compulsiveness.

To begin with, medical knowledge is highly technical and often poorly understood by patients. It is difficult for a patient to be sure a physician has done all she or he can in making a diagnosis or carrying out a treatment. The burden of completeness, therefore, falls on the physician. In addition, physicians are dependent on other physicians and medical technicians for much of their diagnostic information. Unfortunately x-ray and laboratory reports vary greatly in quality, and it is up to the coordinating physician to determine the quality as well as to question the individual results if they fit poorly with the clinical picture. It is also vital to remember that all specific treatments involve the risk of adverse results. Physicians must be convinced that a particular treatment is indicated and must demonstrate continual vigilance to try and prevent or counteract harmful side effects. Finally, a patient's health status changes over time. No single examination or treatment is an end point, and physicians must realize that, whether a patient is well or ill, perpetual and careful reexamination is mandatory. The following example stresses the importance of compulsiveness.

A 60-year-old man presents with pain at the left sternoclavicular junction 6 months following uncomplicated aortic valve replacement. The patient has experienced the usual incisional pain during the immediate postoperative period. However, he says that this particular pain persisted after the general sternal pain disappeared. At this time, it is localized to a small area at the sternoclavicular junction. The pain is slightly aggravated by positional changes, but the area is not tender to touch. The patient has a 40-plus pack-year history of smoking with a morning cough. He reports no increase in severity of the cough and only some greyish sputum. The physician orders a chest x ray with attention to the area in question; it is read as negative. He reassures the patient that this is residual sternal pain secondary to the sternotomy. On a visit 6 months later, the patient complains of the same pain without much change in other symptoms or examination. The physician, a cardiologist used to persistent sternal problems after cardiac surgery, feels comfortable reassuring the patient again that it is residual postoperative sternal pain. No further testing is done. One and one-half years after the symptom began (2 years postoperatively), the patient presents with somewhat worse pain and some swelling over the painful area; at this time, the wife reports hemoptysis. The wife informs the physician that the patient is color-blind and that she suspects he has been coughing up blood for several months. This time, a chest x ray suggests a lung and rib lesion, and chest computed tomography followed by biopsy confirms a small-cell carcinoma of the lung. On review of the first chest x ray, a different radiologist points out a subtle lesion that has been there all along.

This case was subtle, and it is not difficult to see how the diagnosis was missed. However, several aspects are worthy of comment. It turned out to be important that this man was color-blind. No physician had obtained this information. In addition, the cardiologist was quick to accept the usual explanation for chest-wall pain (i.e. postoperative sternal problems). When such a localized and specific complaint persisted, a more compulsive physician might have searched further for other explanations. Although the initial chest x-ray report was negative, the patient continued to complain of the same localized pain for 1.5 years. The physician should have taken the film to other radiologists, repeated the x ray sooner, or obtained special rib views. The more subtle a problem is, the more important compulsiveness can be.

Flexibility has been emphasized less than compulsiveness. The amount of technical knowledge necessary to practice good medicine is vast. Medical education tends to be organized rigidly to facilitate mastery of this material. Yet illness often varies from its textbook description, and the physician must be flexible enough to account for these variations. Since every patient is a unique person, successful delivery of good care demands that patient individuality be appreciated and taken into account in the diagnostic and therapeutic process. An example follows:

A 53-year-old professor with bowel cancer, treated with colectomy and pelvic irradiation 1.5 years ago, comes to the emergency room with a swollen, red, tender leg. She is afebrile. A venogram is negative. The diagnosis appears to be cellulitis. The patient's physician advises hospitalization for intravenous antibiotics. The patient balks because of a lecture she must write for which she needs her home library. The internist is firm. The professor continues to object. Finally, the internist strikes a bargain. She will let her go home if she stays in bed, puts her leg up, takes oral antibiotics and calls early the next day to report. The patient agrees. By the next day, the leg is even more painful, and the professor requests hospitalization. The internist admits a willing, rather than an angry patient.

Such flexibility is not always possible, but when it is, it can help win over a patient. The rapport that follows may have broader implications including the degree to which the patient reports symptoms and side effects and the extent to which the patient complies with future recommendations. In general, if the patient has been led to expect a flexible response, the physician-patient relationship will be much more satisfactory.

Conclusion

It is obvious that we have arbitrarily chosen some highlights of what is often called the art of medicine. This art is something we should continually try to refine over the course of our medical careers. None of us has mastered it; we all need to strive in that direction. The process begins when one realizes the serious responsibility involved in the physician role and when this responsibility is discharged by *caring* for patients as well as for their illnesses. This type of caring is particularly important now that so much technology is employed in medical care. Technical aspects of medical care should not overshadow humanistic elements. Patients should not be subjected to one diagnostic procedure after another without careful explanation of each procedure and without sufficient time between procedures to recover. Physicians should listen to patients rather than just lecture them. Patients should not be embarrassed with personal questions or requests to disrobe in front of an audience. They should not be ignored while the physician carries on conversations with colleagues and staff or addressed as if they were incapable of understanding simple medical explanations. Physicians should not communicate with patients in brief, technical, and confusing sentences, allowing no time for the patients' questions. They should not always remain standing at the bedside, looking down on the patient, instead of at the same level. While a certain inner toughness is an important attribute for a physician, it should not preclude empathy. Physicians should constantly ask themselves, "How would *I feel* if the patient in the bed were me?"

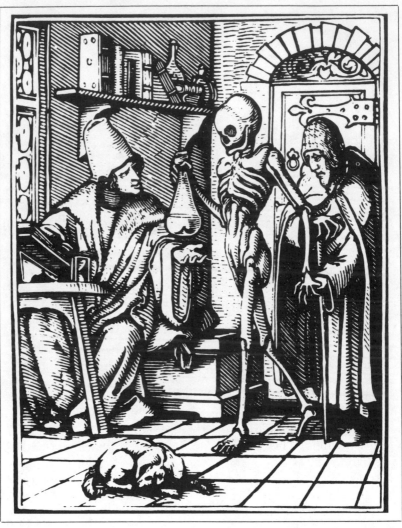

"The Dance of Death." Death confronts the physician with a urine sample from an ailing patient (in the background). The quote below the print stated, "Physician, heal thyself." (A woodcut from Hans Holbein the Younger's series of woodcuts.)

3. Dealing with Burnout

Burnout is a word coined in 1975 to describe a constellation of symptoms of physical, intellectual, and emotional exhaustion in mental health workers (Freudenberger, 1975). The term has since been applied to people in almost any work situation. It implies a kind of "wearing out."

Physicians are at particularly high risk for burnout, partly because of their personalities and partly because of the demands made on them. Like most problems, burnout is better prevented than rectified. Yet medical school admissions committees do not try to identify those with a predisposition for it, and little mention of the problem is made during medical school or in postgraduate training. In fact, medical education appears to be designed to facilitate its occurrence.

Many things attract people to medicine: intellectual interest, opportunity for significant service to other people, comfortable income, status, power. These goals can all be achieved without suffering burnout. However, the idealized image of the physician held by the public and the physician's compulsive attempts to live up to the image may sow some of the seeds of this syndrome.

Young people first encounter a physician as a magic figure who is often accompanied by discomfort in one form or another. Curiously enough, physicians are appreciated, even revered, for inflicting these hardships. This places doctors in the category of priests, kings, and great warriors: wonderful role models for the young to aspire to as they struggle with the helplessness of their early years. Little happens to change this image as people grow up. Adults retain this romantic picture, even embellish it. Robert Louis Stevenson wrote:

"There are men and classes of men that stand above the common herd: the soldier, the sailor, and the shepherd not infrequently; the artist rarely; rarelier still the clergyman; the physician almost as a rule. He is the flower (such as it is) of our civilization; . . . Generosity he has, such as is possible to those who practice an art, . . . discretion, tested by a hundred secrets; tact, tried in a thousand embarrassments; and what are more important, Heraclean cheerfulness and courage." (Chandler, 1983)

This idealized role is expected of the physician by the public and often demanded by the physician of her- or himself. Given this expectation, it is little wonder that persons with a very great need for approval aspire to be physicians. Given this image, it is no less mysterious that the physician's professional training is characterized by great physical, intellectual, and emotional demands. The unwritten assumption during training is that to be worthy of a medical degree, one must master volumes of technical material, withstand chronic fatigue without impairment, and meet difficult emotional situations without suffering. What happens when this romantic projection goes awry? The following example illustrates what can happen to even a young physician in a system that sees itself as elite, demanding, and single-minded.

A 32-year-old medical resident rushes into the conference room at 10:45 A.M. for attending rounds, which began at 10:30. She reaches for her clipboard and realizes she does not have it. She must have left it in the nurses' station as she rushed off. The attending comments on her lateness. The resident begins to recount her bad night but stops as she realizes that no one is interested. She begins to present a case but is interrupted by a page, which she nervously answers while everyone stares at her. After the case presentation, she is asked several questions about the pathophysiology of the patient's illness. Her answers are not too clear. At the end of rounds, the attending physician pulls her aside and says, "You know, I realize you're busy but you're going to have to learn to do three things at once, do them well, and be on time. When I was a resident, we were on call every other night, and our discussions were expected to be letter-perfect." The resident flushes, feels the anger well up inside her, but does not speak. A nurse hails her about a patient who cannot void. "I'll get to it," she snaps, as she walks off down the hall.

This young physician already illustrates a life pattern that is bound to produce burnout. She is *overcommitted,* at least for her abilities, and *exhausted.* Thus, she is perpetually late, often forgets things, and never feels completely in control of the situation. Even her medical thinking begins to slip. This leads to guilt feelings on her part and chastisement by others. She is denied the approval she so much wants. Her training has emphasized retention of facts, rigidity of protocols, toughness, compulsiveness, and deference to authority, rather than the exercise of reason, flexibility, introspection, and assertiveness; she is likely to respond by working even harder, becoming even more exhausted, and failing even more noticeably rather than by stopping to examine the problem and planning her life more carefully.

Since the demands made on her by patients and nurses carry less clout than those of attending physicians, it is towards the first two that she will vent her *frustration, irritability, cynicism,* even *an-*

ger. Thus, we note the scenario of the resident walking off down the hall instead of tending to the patient who could not void. As she ignores this patient, the young physician risks destroying *her most important resource, her commitment to patient care.*

"The foundation of good medical care is giving a damn; most of us already know how to practice far better medicine than we do. Usually, when I don't do as well by a particular patient as I might have, the primary obstacle is *me:* my lack of interest or enthusiasm or energy. . . . My satisfaction from the process tends to diminish proportionately, and something unsavory happens to my self-respect as well." (Lipp, 1977)

If one survives and graduates from this system, one is ill prepared to face the demands of medical practice. These demands are great. Some are different from training, others are the same. Among the differences is a change in role. One is no longer the trainee. One is the attending physician. With this new authority may come the problem of running the business of a medical practice with all its complexities, including increasing competition and increasing governmental and insurance intervention. If one chooses academic medicine, there is pressure to obtain grants, to publish, and to produce some practice income while pursuing academic goals. Even if one avoids both of these roles by working for a large group practice, there are still the pressures engendered by patient care.

These pressures are many and range from compelling to trivial. Among the more compelling are *decisions clouded by ambiguity.* Have I done enough studies to exclude a serious illness? Do I have enough information to make a particular diagnosis? Does the potential gain from a particular treatment outweigh the risk of a serious side effect? Can I perform a particular procedure without causing the patient significant pain or harm? Simultaneously with the ambiguities, one must deal with *emotionally draining encounters:* the death of a patient, the grief of the patient's family, the need to deliver bad news and to help the family absorb the shock and deal with the pain, the necessity of watching suffering without being able to alleviate it adequately, the tension involved in dealing with issues of sexuality. The ambiguous decisions and the emotional encounters do not come in an orderly fashion, one at a time, properly spaced. More often they occur rapidly, repetitively, relentlessly. As if this is not enough, there are more aggravating intrusions. Patients may be angry if they are not improving, whether or not it is the physician's fault. Patients may want to be seen immediately, no matter how minor the problem. Patients may interrupt the handling of a serious problem with the report of a more trivial problem, using the phrase "I thought you'd want to know." And so on, and so on, and so on.

In the beginning, the physician often has the energy needed to grapple with this panorama of demands. However, *if self-expectations are too high, if involvement is too complete, if ability to plan is poor,* a wearing-out process begins. The symptoms of this process include a feeling of harassment, an overlay of irritability, a cynical manner, exaggerated hopes of satisfaction from financial gain or material things at times, depression, and even a resort to drugs or alcohol at other times. The following scenario depicts a physician in the late stages of burnout.

It is 12:45 P.M. A group of attending physicians are having lunch in the physicians' dining room. Dr. A says, "Sometimes I wonder if it's worth it nowadays. My desk is buried in forms; all my patients think they're the only sick person in the city, and all I read about is malpractice suits and how DRGs are going to screw the practicing physician." Dr. B answers, "I know! I've got to get away. I bought this condominium in Vermont. My family is going to be there for a week around the holidays, and I'm going to try to grab a day up there. Damn! It's 1:15 already! By the time I get to the office, I'll start a half-hour behind."

Dr. B drives to his office. As he walks through the door, one of his medical assistants rushes up and says, "Mr. Z has been waiting since one o'clock, and he's threatening to leave if he has to wait any longer." Another of the office staff says, "Could you call Ms. Y as soon as you can? She's in terrible pain! And can you see the drug representative from company X for a minute? She says she's tried five times to see you." Just then the physician's beeper rings. As he looks down at his cluttered desk, he sees the list of afternoon patients. "Oh no!" he thinks as he looks at the second name—a very demanding patient. He reaches into his desk, pulls out a physician's sample of diazepam, takes 5 mg, and turns to face the afternoon.

After struggling through 15 office patients, nine phone calls, and some paper work between 1:30 and 5:30, Dr. B drives back to the hospital for a new admission, a consultation, and two sick patients. He knows he will not be home before 7:30, but at least the chaos of the afternoon is over. In the coatroom, he picks up the phone to call home. He is a little nervous each time he has to call home to say he will be late, although this happens three to four times a week. In one of the nurses' stations, a nurse commiserates with him about having to work late again. When Dr. B is finally finished, he is very tired. He thinks about the drink waiting at home. He is nervous about the reception he will get at home when he walks in even later than anticipated.

This physician is overcommitted, perpetually late, frustrated, isolated, depressed, and substance-dependent. What little satisfaction he obtains comes from trading complaints with colleagues, drawing sympathy from hospital personnel—sympathy he does not get at home—and dreaming or talking about material things that he has too little time to enjoy. How can this scenario be avoided?

The answer may well begin with medical school admissions policies. Potential physicians should have a truly broad education. Once they enter medicine, it would be helpful to them to develop an interest in the arts, literature, philosophy, skills in sports, hobbies. This would provide a much-needed outlet from medicine. Medical school admissions committees might also look for people who are capable of managing their time. This might predict adeptness at handling the myriad demands of the profession.

In medical school, students should be encouraged to take care of themselves as well as their patients. Policemen, firemen, and deep-sea divers are educated in the dangers of their professions. They are taught survival techniques. Physicians should be similarly taught. Among the survival strategies should be the avoidance of burnout. At present, instead of anticipating and trying to prevent this problem, the stage is set for it. "By asking students to care about their patients without caring about themselves these programs create an impossible dilemma in physicians' later lives" (Hamburg, 1982).

In order to avoid burnout, one must find satisfaction in both work and home life. Since medicine is stimulating and since physicians are generally intelligent and learned, there should be no problem in finding satisfaction with work. Yet there often is a problem. If we had to choose one reason, it would be poor planning, leading to *inadequate time* for care of individual patients, for keeping abreast of medical advances, and for absorbing unexpected problems. Physicians need to *plan* their activities. They need to leave enough time to do a high-quality job that will bring them satisfaction. They need to leave enough time for learning and growth. They need to leave *unscheduled time* for the unexpected. They must learn to *anticipate* rather than exhibit merely *responsive behavior*. To do this, they must *set limits.*

Physicians must also realize that a satisfying home life requires adequate time. Family and friends need attention, interest, and support. Some medical marriages have been described as "living alone with someone." This situation inevitably leads to strife. Family provides support only if it receives support.

Physicians need outlets other than medicine. If one is single-minded, one gradually loses perspective. Professional disappointments become overwhelming instead of being balanced by satisfactions in other areas. Nonmedical matters gradually become remote until one almost fears to encounter them. This causes quiet isolation at best and too often anger at being excluded. Oliver Wendell Holmes said:

"The longer I live, the more I am satisfied of two things: first, that the truest lives are those that are cut rose-diamond fashion with many facets answering to the many-planed aspects of the world about them, secondly, that society is always trying in some way or other to grind us down to a single flat surface. It is hard work to resist this grinding-down action." (Chandler, 1983)

Finally, some physicians need *periodic changes in professional emphasis.* Any job, no matter how complex, becomes routine after a great deal of repetition. Change may supply the challenge that has dissipated over the years. A generalist may choose to focus more on some specialty that she or he likes. A specialist may decide to become more of a generalist. A clinician may elect to take on more administrative duties. Some physicians even turn from medicine to another career. The point is that *change introduces challenge.*

Burnout is not a theoretic problem: It is widespread. It converts intelligent, motivated, sensitive physicians into impaired, disgruntled, inconsiderate ones. The waste of talent and knowledge is dismaying. The consequent suffering of both physicians and patients is tragic. At present, the problem of burnout appears to be confronted most often after the fact, at a time when a great deal of damage has already been done. It should be anticipated.

Suggested Reading

Chandler, E. T. *The Creative Physician.* In J. P. Callan (ed.), *The Physician: A Professional Under Stress.* Norwalk, Conn.: Appleton-Century-Crofts, 1983.

Freudenberger, H. J. The staff burn-out syndrome in alternative institutions. *Psychotherapeutic Theory Res. Pract.* 12:73, 1975.

Hamburg, P. Letter to the editor. *N. Engl. J. Med.* 307:563, 1982.

Lipp, M. R. *Respectful Treatment, The Human Side of Medical Care.* Hagerstown, Md.: Harper & Row, 1977. P. 206.

Pepper, T. H. Physician burnout: Avoiding being your own worst arsonist. *W. Va. Med. J.* 78:184, 1982.

Vincent, M. O. Some sequelae of stress in physicians. *Psychiatr. J. Univ. Ottawa* 8:120, 1983.

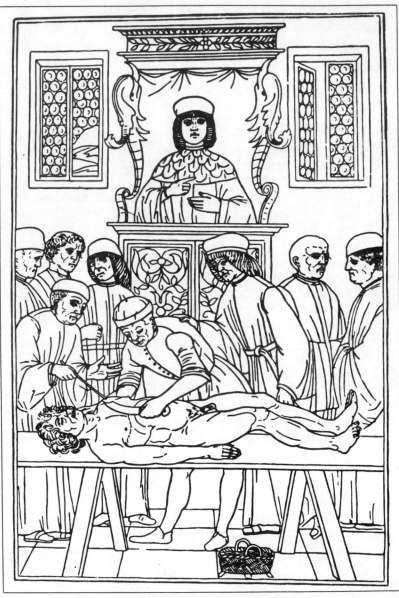

A Renaissance anatomy lesson: The professor sits above it all, expounding, while a prosector performs the dissection.

4. Medical Traditions and Current Challenges in the Delivery of Medical Care

Medical students and young physicians often wonder about the value of understanding medical history and the traditions of medical care in earlier periods. Harassed by an ever-growing avalanche of scientific and technologic information, today's young physicians and medical students feel, with some justification, that it is impossible to know everything. Therefore, why not sacrifice a superficial knowledge, at best, of medical care and traditions in past decades and centuries? The purpose of this chapter is twofold: to review medical traditions that can be useful in our times and to examine the challenges of delivering humane and humanistic medical care in the waning years of the twentieth century.

Reassurance and Encouragement

An extensive knowledge of medical history is not necessary in order to gain a perspective on today's medical practice. A brief review of earlier centuries provides a clear picture of inaccuracy in diagnosis and ineffectiveness in therapy. The only positive therapeutic aspects of medical care for many hundreds of years were the kindness, empathy, and concern of the physician for the patient. The application of these personal qualities resulted in improved clinical status for some patients and decreased fear and anxiety in many individuals. The improvement observed in selected patients was probably the result of a beneficial process initiated by confidence in the physician and expectations of improvement—that is, the placebo effect (see Chaps. 2,11), which can lead to increased endorphin levels in the central nervous system. A current counterpart of this beneficial effect can be observed daily in intensive care units of most modern hospitals: Fear, anxiety, pain, and even arrhythmias are often ameliorated through the ministrations of a caring and thoughtful nurse. Even potentially life-threatening situations can be markedly improved by such gentle and kind attention to the patient.

An elderly woman with severe respiratory distress secondary to pulmonary edema is gently "talked out" of her condition by an experienced physician, using very small dosages of intravenous morphine together with kind words and a caring approach. The physician administers a small dosage of intravenous morphine while simultaneously suggesting to the patient that she is in good hands, that she will soon feel less short of breath, and that she can relax and breathe more deeply and slowly. Within a few minutes, the patient's respiratory rate is nearly normal, and she is markedly less anxious.

It is likely that the mechanism of these beneficial responses was decreased activation of the sympathetic nervous system with resultant drops in heart rate and systemic blood pressure.

The Reality of Death

Another lesson that can be learned from medical tradition is a sense of what can and what cannot be achieved in medical practice. All living things must die at some point. Despite the remarkable scientific and technologic mechanisms available for clinical practice, there comes a point when the burden of disease on a particular patient is so great that the individual dies. This state of affairs has existed throughout recorded and unrecorded medical history; physicians have been forced to learn how to deal with it. We must help both our patients and ourselves face this most difficult of all human trials.

At times, dealing with impending death can be very trying for the modern physician, who is trained to "win the battle" against death. Physicians in earlier periods accepted human mortality as an inevitable event. Less tension and frustration were aroused since death was the expected outcome. The modern physician must learn to deal with death as his or her predecessors were forced to. Having learned to cope personally with this final, unavoidable outcome, the physician *must* endeavor to aid and support the patient and the grieving family as well. Many approaches are effective in these circumstances. All techniques have the following characteristics in common: serious affect (do not make light of the patient's symptoms), warmth and concern, willingness to answer questions, and supportive reassurance.

Modern patients frequently have unrealistic expectations with respect to anticipated miracles on the part of the physician. When such remarkable cures are not forthcoming, patients and family members may become distant, cold, and even openly hostile to the physician. In such circumstances, and even earlier in the clinical course, it is important for the physician to educate the patient and his or her family *gently* concerning realistic expectations. Answering questions with patience and candor will usually ameliorate the situation, thereby decreasing further anxiety and hostility.

Indeed, such communication is also of considerable benefit in patients for whom effective medical or surgical therapy is available. One should not ignore the potential synergistic effect of lowered anxiety and discomfort added to an effective therapeutic program. Efficacious therapy is further improved by a positive psychologic atmosphere.

Discussing Risk

An analogous situation arises when the physician seeks the patient's permission to perform a potentially risky or arduous diagnostic or therapeutic procedure. It can easily be understood that patients and family members dread such interventions. Frequently, physicians err in their approach to patients under such circumstances: Potential complications and the risk of dying are presented to the patient without explanation. The result is an increased sense of anxiety in the patient and family members.

Following an extensive diagnostic evaluation, an internist advises aortic valve replacement for an elderly man with critical aortic stenosis. A surgeon is consulted, who presents the patient with a strictly factual assessment of the risk of the planned surgery. The patient becomes distraught and contemplates refusing the projected operation. The internist reviews the potential risks of surgery with the patient, interpreting the numbers and showing the patient that such untoward and unpleasant outcomes are decidedly *less likely* than a smooth operative and postoperative course and that the *expected* outcome is favorable despite the potential risks. The patient accepts the risks and undergoes elective aortic valve replacement.

As this example demonstrates, there are two ways to present bad news to a patient: the overly candid and somewhat cruel technique of stating risks of mortality and morbidity as if one were reading a grocery list and the more humanistic method of mentioning potential risks but at the same time explaining that these are unusual or unanticipated outcomes. Kindness and empathy are essential qualities in a physician: The patient is not contemplating replacing the carburetor on his or her car. On the contrary, the person sitting across from the physician is pondering personal discomfort and even mortality.

Primum non nocere:
First, Do No Harm

This ancient medical paradigm is Hippocratic in origin. It stems from an epoch when physicians had little other than psychologic support and kindness to offer patients. In the latter half of the twentieth century, when effective diagnostic and therapeutic interventions are commonplace, it is a commonly forgotten dictum. Patients, however, have not changed in the 2500 years since Hippocrates was alive. Their fears and anxieties are just as palpable today as in earlier eras. The physician must weigh the potential harm of a procedure or a therapeutic strategy before offering it to the patient. If little benefit can be anticipated from a particular course of action, it should not be presented to the patient as an option: *primum non nocere.* The following example illustrates this dictum:

A chronically ill patient with metastatic adenocarcinoma of the pancreas develops total biliary obstruction. The physician realizes that this complication will be fatal if aggressive diagnostic and therapeutic interventions are not performed expeditiously. However, the physician also realizes that relief of biliary obstruction in this patient will lead to only a few weeks or months of painful, agonizing survival. In the tradition of *primum non nocere,* the patient is treated with analgesics, and aggressive diagnostic and therapeutic interventions are withheld.

Of course, *primum non nocere* should *not* be interpreted as "do nothing" (i.e., diagnostic and therapeutic nihilism for all patients). It merely suggests that the physician contemplate anticipated benefits weighed against potential risks before initiating a course of action in a particular individual.

High Technology in Medicine

Recent decades have been filled with extraordinary technologic advances in medicine, including computerized x ray, nuclear magnetic resonance imaging, and even laser therapy. Such technologic developments have greatly increased the physician's diagnostic and therapeutic abilities. Even the most occult malignancies can now be visualized and treated by a variety of innovative techniques. Occluded blood vessels can be reopened and destroyed joints replaced. Unfortunately, nonmedical people are often ambiguous in their response to such technical advances. While acknowledging these improvements in diagnosis and therapy, such individuals decry the alienation and removal of the physician from the patient's bedside that may result from technical developments. The physician is seen as an evil scientist, following in the footsteps of Dr. Frankenstein or Dr. Jekyll and Mr. Hyde, exploring new scientific paths instead of aiding and supporting the patient. It is not uncommon to hear patients in large tertiary care centers complain of being experimented on even when routine diagnostic and therapeutic strategies are employed. These individuals have failed to understand that in some situations the only way to arrive at a beneficial therapeutic program is through trial and error. Instead, they observe that their physician is increasingly involved with computerized diagnostic and therapeutic equipment and less involved with them as human beings. Some physicians support this perception by their cold and distant approach to patients. The image of the medical profession is being altered by these forces: No longer is the physician seen as the warm, caring, and supportive individual of housecall days. Rather, he or she is thought of as a technician, operating complex machinery without concern for the human beings placed at the mercy of these seemingly malevolent instruments of technology.

How can we reverse this insidious and detrimental degradation of our image as humane healers and supporters? Again, it is crucial to understand that such negative images result when physicians fail to communicate with patients. Even highly complex and massive machinery can be presented to patients in a manner that eliminates fear and anxiety aroused by such devices. Recognition of the patient's fears and a warm and friendly explanation of the positive aspects of such technologic instrumentation invariably achieves the hoped-for result: "This device will enable us to take a kind of photograph of your liver in order to see if that is what is causing your discomfort." "This equipment enables us to see where the blockages are in your blood vessels so that we can repair them and help you feel better." These are just two of the many ways that complex machinery can be explained to patients, thereby eliminating the fear associated with these technologic instruments. Careful, friendly, supportive explanation by the physician concerning every diagnostic and therapeutic intervention is the only route to elimination of the "mad scientist" image associated with the use of high technology in medical care. Videotapes explaining procedures such as cardiac catheterization are also very helpful in reducing patient anxiety. Some nurses in coronary care units describe the extensive monitoring equipment and procedures to patients as "electronic guardian angels," again stressing the positive, nonthreatening nature of the technology.

Finally, it is important to point out to patients that *concerned human beings* are in control of all the technical equipment employed for diagnosis and therapy. The patient is *not* being turned over to a computerized robot that performs its task without regard to the patient's physical or psychologic discomfort. Such equipment is directed and controlled by human beings interested in the patient's well-being. Physicians should be alert to the potential for patient discomfort before, during, and after diagnostic investigation. A common example is the prolonged wait many patients experience in drafty hallways before and after a procedure.

As soon as results of tests or therapeutic procedures are available, they should be discussed with the patient, again stressing how the technical device assisted the physician in making the appropriate diagnostic or therapeutic decision. In this manner, patients are relieved of the misconception that the equipment itself is making decisions that affect morbidity and mortality. High technology should be presented as an *aid* to decision making by the physician, not as the prime mover of that process.

Medical Economics

There are extraordinary economic forces at work today in medicine. Medical care costs have increased greatly since the mid-1960s, spawning a number of different schemes for physician and hospital reimbursement. The spread of prepaid health plans in which patients (and often their employers) pay a fixed yearly sum for all in- and outpatient health services is exerting a considerable influence on medical economics since administrators for such plans seek to deliver medical care at the lowest cost. Competition among hospitals and physicians for patients as well as pressure from prepaid health care plans is forcing providers of medical care to reassess their billing procedures, their efficiency, and their fee structure. The remaining years of the twentieth century will witness increasingly severe pressure on the medical profession to hold down costs and increase service.

In this economic climate, a number of health care planners and administrators have devised medical care delivery systems that resemble those employed in durable good industries. Patients are considered products or service recipients, while physicians are compared with factories or service facilities. Although such economic plans can hold down medical care costs, there are inherent problems in such models.

Patients are not comparable to soft drinks, cars, or food products. Indeed, strict business efficiency applied to health care can foster distance and indifference between physician and patient. Illness is such a personal occurrence, fraught with discomfort and anxiety, that physicians cannot treat patients as if they were products on an assembly line. Personal warmth, careful explanation, and human contact are vital to the relationship between doctor and patient (see Chap. 2). Such a relationship cannot be developed if medical care is delivered in assembly line fashion.

Cost-containment schemes, seeking to control medical care expenses, must take the very personal nature of the doctor-patient relationship into account. Excessive efficiency in the delivery of health care can have a negative influence on medical care. Kindness, empathy, and compassion must not be sacrificed to economic expediency. As noted earlier, patients do not want to be treated as if they were machines or merely insignificant cogs in a giant, computerized schema. Patients want a personal relationship with their physicians; the more depersonalized medical care becomes, the greater patient unhappiness will be. Although medicine in the United States will probably never return to the style of the house-call era, loss of close human contact between doctor and patient will lead to irreparable deterioration in the quality of medical care. The humanistic element in medicine is as important as high-technology diagnostic and therapeutic intervention. The key to delivery of excellent medical care cannot be summarized better than by Dr. F. W. Peabody, who stated, "The secret of the care of the patient is in caring for the patient" (Peabody, 1959).

Suggested Reading

Blumgart, H. L. Caring for the patient. *N. Engl. J. Med.* 270:449, 1964.
Peabody, F. W. Care of patient. *J.A.M.A.* 88:877, 1959.
Tumulty, P. A. What is a clinician and what does he do? *N. Engl. J. Med.* 283:20, 1970.

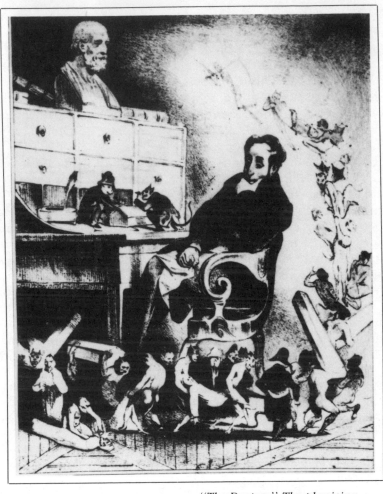

"The Doctor." The physician muses, "How the devil does it happen that all my patients succumb? . . . Yet I bleed them, I purge them, I drug them . . . I simply can't understand!" (Lithograph by Honoré Daumier, 1808–1879.)

5. The Caring Chart

The medical chart serves two functions: During a particular illness, it is a *vehicle for communication among members of the medical care team,* and after the patient leaves the hospital, it becomes *a permanent record of the patient's interaction with the medical care system.* In the performance of these functions, it may serve the patient well or ill, reflecting favorably or unfavorably on the actions and communications of the medical team. Physicians spend a great part of their lives (at times too much) writing and reading charts. It behooves them to spend this time well for the sake of their patients and themselves. This chapter discusses several characteristics that help promote this goal.

Availability
To be used, charts must be available. In many hospitals, especially large teaching hospitals, almost as much time is spent locating charts as writing and reading them. Charts are used by floor secretaries, nurses, attending physicians, medical students, social workers, dieticians, various technicians (e.g., x ray, electrocardiogram [ECG]), various therapists (e.g., respiratory, rehabilitation), and sometimes, hospital administrators. Charts are taken to the nurses' station, conference rooms, patients' rooms, and testing areas. Some responsibility must be taken by all those who handle charts for providing information about where they can be found and for returning them to some central location such as the chart rack. We suggest some color-coded signal system over each chart slot, identifying one of several possible locations (e.g., in nurses' station, in physicians' room, in nurses' charting room, in patient's room, off floor). We also suggest following a variant of the golden rule: *Return the chart after using it since others abhor the chart hunt as much as you do.*

Readability
To be useful, charts must be readable. Even though legibility does not correlate with ability, performance of medical tasks, or concern for the patient, legibility is mandatory if the chart is to be useful for present communications or future reference. Thus, physicians

should do whatever is required to improve legibility: Write more slowly, print, type, or just try harder to bring their particular handwriting up to a decipherable level. *We must all be visibly intolerant of illegible chart entries.*

Abbreviations are so ingrained in medical writing that it is unrealistic to speak out against them. However, physicians must make some effort to limit their use and to use standardized abbreviations. The following example is an abuse of abbreviations:

57 y.o. ♂ S/P AAA op dvp'd AMI c̄ CHF & CHB.

This description loses any sense of the patient who is its subject. In addition, one of the abbreviations is unclear. Is AMI anterior myocardial infarction or acute myocardial infarction? We would plead for some compromise such as

57 y.o. man S/P abdominal aortic aneurysm repair developed an anterior MI complicated by CHF and complete heart block.

Publications like the *Medical Abbreviations Handbook* may be helpful to check if abbreviations are acceptable.

Understandability

Charts are generally organized into sections such as history and physical examination, progress notes, and laboratory work. Two sections that are crucial to good patient care are the *problem list* (often placed in the front of the chart) and the *medication list*. The problem list is written and maintained by the physician. It should be executed in bold and legible script. Active problems must be clearly separated from inactive ones, with dating when possible. The medication list is generally written and updated by the nursing or clerical staff. It is the physician's responsibility to check its accuracy. Both of these lists *must be updated one or more times per day*. Physicians should go through both lists carefully each time they write a note in the chart. This will minimize mistakes in patient care.

Information placed in the chart should be precise. One frequently sees vague entries that leave questions in the chart reader's mind. Some examples follow:

a. Family history strongly positive.

b. Patient has had two previous MIs.
c. Patient has had an ulcer.

These would be better if they read

a. Family history strongly positive for CAD with father dying age 49 of MI and brother undergoing triple CABG at age 53.
b. Patient had an anterior Q wave MI 5 years ago and an inferior non-Q wave MI 3 years ago.
c. Patient had x-ray-proven gastric ulcer 3 years ago with no problems since then.

Progress notes should be written utilizing some accepted system. The most popular one at present is taken from Weed's *The Problem Oriented Record* (Weed, 1969) and goes by the acronym *SOAP* (subjective, objective, assessment, and plan). *Entries must be separate for different problems.* An example follows:

DIABETES
S   Patient is less thirsty.
O   Skin turgor is improved; fasting blood sugar is decreased from 420 to 180.
A   Hyperglycemia is resolving.
P   Begin maintenance insulin with NPH tomorrow at 40 units per day.

CONGESTIVE HEART FAILURE
S   Patient is breathing more comfortably.
O   Lungs are now clear; S3 gallop is gone.
A   CHF is resolving.
P   Begin oral furosemide tomorrow at 40 mg per day.

All active problems should be updated daily. However, inactive ones need not be mentioned. *There is a fine line between a complete and a verbose chart.* It is helpful to *resummarize the problem every few days* for those who have not been following it as closely as the primary physician. The following example refers back to the previous example.

CONGESTIVE HEART FAILURE
Day 5 following large anterior MI complicated by CHF
S   Patient is breathing more comfortably.

O   Lungs are now clear; S3 gallop is gone.
A   CHF is resolving.
P   Begin oral furosemide tomorrow at 40 mg per day.

When recording procedures, it is helpful to highlight them so that another person need not hunt for them when reviewing the chart. In addition, one should include all the data pertinent to the procedure. An example follows:

CARDIOVERSION NOTE

Indication	Atrial flutter with ventricular rate 150 per minute.
Anesthesia	IV valium 12 mg.
Energy	50 Wsec, 100 Wsec, 200 Wsec.
Result	NSR after the third shock.
Complications	None.
Medication	Continue digoxin 0.125 mg per day and quinidine sulfate 300 mg 4 times per day.

Reliability

Chart entries should obviously be accurate. *In order to ensure accuracy, it is necessary to record precisely what happened.* A vague note may lead to a misinterpretation and improper treatment. The following example illustrates this:

A 73-year-old woman is in the hospital because her angina pectoris has been poorly controlled as an outpatient. One evening she complains of chest pain. The nurse gives her a nitroglycerin with equivocal relief, and the covering house officer is called. By the time he gets there, she is fairly comfortable and does not require additional medication. On questioning, he learns that the pain she has had is aggravated by deep breathing and is unlike her anginal pain. He is rushed, and in his note, he writes only "episode of chest pain—patient now comfortable and with normal vital signs." On rounds the next morning, the patient's regular physicians do not query her about the previous night's pain since the covering physician's note raises no questions. They simply ask her if she has had any further episodes. Even though she says no, they decide to increase her antianginal medication since her pain is not completely controlled.

In this example, the regular physicians did not appreciate the pleuritic nature of the pain, and thus, they treated her inappropriately and failed to follow up on the pleuritic symptoms. The covering house officer could have prevented this by giving a more precise description of her symptoms.

Physicians' notes should be consistent with and often include references to nurses' notes. In some hospitals, physicians and nurses write on the same page. When this occurs, some joint agreement about uniform abbreviations must be made. The physician sees the patient relatively briefly. The nursing staff interacts with the patient multiple times during the day. Nurses' notes can give the physician valuable information. For example, the nurses might describe intermittent pain or confusion that the patient does not report. Conversely, they may describe a patient as comfortable most of the time despite the fact that the patient complains of discomfort each time the physician is in the room. Nurses may report important psychosocial data such as an argument between the patient and a family member during a visit. To wit, careful reading of nurses' notes is important for delivering good patient care. It is also essential for medical and legal purposes. When charts are reviewed by lawyers in malpractice cases, nurses' notes are scrutinized very carefully.

A 57-year-old man with terminal congestive heart failure decides to make some alterations in his will. He dies soon afterward. One member of his family disputes the will. His physician, who has known him for years, knows that the changes were well thought out and that they reflected the patient's feelings. During the trial, the physician takes the witness stand and testifies in favor of the patient's competence. The lawyer for the disputing family member says, "Doctor, you have told the court that the patient was fully competent when he changed his will. Is that correct?" "Yes," the physician answers. The lawyer then hands the physician a copy of the medical record from the day the patient had executed the change in the will. This includes the nurses' notes, which the physician has not read. The lawyer for the disputing family member than says, "Doctor, would you please read to the court from the nurses' notes? Begin with the entry marked 2:15 P.M." The physician begins to read. "Patient ate only a small part of his lunch. When I went in to remove his tray and later again when I went in to give him medication, he seemed intermittently confused."

The physician was stunned and dismayed. His own notes from that and the next day made no mention of his patient's mental status. Had he routinely read the nurses' notes, he might have commented on those observations in his note. At the very least, he would have known about the observation and thus not been surprised at the trial.

Physicians' orders should reflect their progress notes. Similarly, the progress notes should explain the orders. This is especially important when the dose of a medication is changed or a new medication is added. It might even be useful to highlight major medication changes in a manner similar to that suggested earlier for procedures. This would vastly facilitate chart review. An example follows:

HYPERTENSION
S   Asymptomatic.
O   BP 180/100 supine and standing.
A   Hypertension not well controlled on diuretic alone.
P   Add CAPTOPRIL *12.5 mg 3 times per day* 1 hour before meals.

Someone scanning the chart later would have no trouble following the sequence of medication changes. Presumably, an order for the captopril would appear in the order sheet on the corresponding date.

Humanistic Considerations
Physicians must never forget that a chart is a record of a *person's illness.* In this era of sophisticated technology, it is easy to lose a person's individuality amid the array of technical entries. Several things may help avoid this. First, psychosocial data must be included in the chart. Although much of this information will go in the social history, inclusion of some psychosocial data in other parts of the chart will personalize the record. For example, the present illness might read like this:

This 57-year-old man, who teaches history at a university, was admitted with severe chest pain. The patient has been under a good deal of emotional stress recently because of a grant deadline. On the night of admission, he developed severe, persistent, substernal pain. . .

In a few sentences, we have obtained a picture of a person as opposed to "just another MI." As this patient's hospitalization progresses, other humanistic problems may develop (i.e., anxiety, insomnia, nightmares). These should not be forgotten as one writes daily progress notes. If the SOAP method is being used, and one is not sure where to put such entries, one could use a general category.

GENERAL
S   Patient complains of restlessness.
O   Patient shifts around continually in bed; asks many questions such as "Will I be able to drive? Will I be able to chop wood?"

A   Anxiety over the consequences of the MI.

P   Explain the MI to the patient including cardiac rehabilitation and the fact that most people return to a normal life style; mild tranquilizers if necessary.

Terms used in chart entries and the *tone set* influence not only how others who read the chart will view the patient, but how we as physicians and human beings think about that patient. Using *dignified terms* where possible and conveying a *respectful tone* remind us to approach the patient with respect and set the stage for others to do the same thing. Similarly, *empathetic terms* may be helpful in patient care. One could say "Ms. X has insomnia." or "Ms. X suffers from insomnia." Using the latter terminology may favorably influence our own and other people's approaches to Ms. X's problem.

When patient and physician talk behind closed doors, it is not difficult for the physician to *honor the patient's right to confidentiality.* When a patient enters the hospital, a complete record of the medical history and at least some references to the patient's psychosocial history are available in open-book form in the middle of the nurses' station. Anyone with access to the area has access to the chart. Since external control of charts going in and out of the chart rack is difficult, physicians must take steps to try and promote privacy. *They should not write material that might seriously embarrass or legally compromise the patient in the chart* (e.g., such things as extramarital affairs or illegal business practices). In addition, physicians should not discuss the patient's illness or private life in open areas with noninvolved bystanders. Finally, physicians must refrain from reading charts, unless they are helping in the patient's care or are asked to read the chart by the patient. They should have no more inclination to read such a chart than they would have to open another person's mail. *It behooves the physician to set standards of confidentiality for other hospital personnel.*

Sometimes, medical personnel disagree with one another about the patient's history, physical examination, pathophysiology, or treatment. The chart should not become a battleground among physicians, nurses, and other providers of health care. Additions, deletions, and different interpretations can be written into the chart with tact and with sensitivity to other people's feelings. Such exchanges as "no S3 gallop heard," followed in the next note by "definite S3 gallop heard" are not necessary. The latter person could have written, "I thought I was able to hear a third sound but will listen again together with (prior physician)." *Humanistic con-*

siderations in the chart should be present among the staff as well.

In summary, we have tried to point out some ways to increase the *availability, readability, understandability, reliability, and humanistic considerations of the medical record.* Most of us will never have a formal biography written of our lives. All of us have or will have medical records written about us. We would like these to be helpful in our care, empathetic to our suffering, and respectful of our individuality. This can be accomplished if all physicians try to produce a *caring chart.*

Suggested Reading

Medical Abbreviations Handbook. Oradell, N. J.: Medical Economics, 1982.
Weed, L. L. *Medical Records, Medical Education and Patient Care.* Cleveland: Case Western Reserve, 1969.

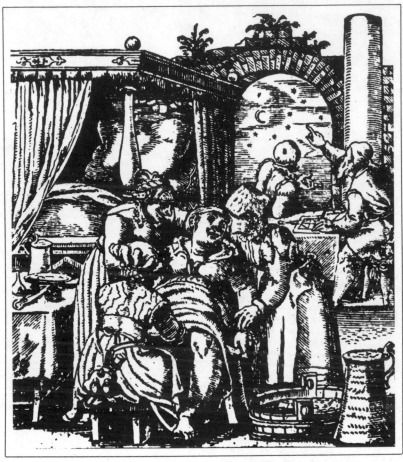

*Renaissance childbirth. The pro-
spective mother sits fully clothed
on a "birthing stool" supported
by two women assistants, while a
midwife delivers the child. The
two physicians in attendance examine the heavens to determine
the astrologic character and future of the expected child.*

6. Continuing Medical Education: Dealing with the Knowledge Explosion

Perhaps no profession except tax law or accounting requires the same attention to continuing postgraduate education as medicine does. It has been estimated that a current graduate of medical school will find his or her education obsolete in 7 years if no attempt is made to follow advances in the field. This is not a new phenomenon. Sir William Osler recognized this fact at the turn of the century at a time when medical research and the volume of medical publication were modest in comparison with current levels:

" . . . [the recent medical graduate] may feel such a relief after graduation that the effort to take to his books is beyond his mental strength, and a weekly journal with an occasional textbook furnish pabulum enough, at least, to keep his mind hibernating. But ten years later he is dead mentally. . . . I would urge him to start at any rate with the books. . . . A good weekly and a good monthly journal to begin with, and read them . . . and as your practice increases, make a habit of buying a few special monographs every year. Read with two objects: first to acquaint yourself with the current knowledge on a subject and the steps by which it has been reached; and secondly, and more important, read to understand and analyse your cases. . . . Every fifth year, back to the hospital, back to the laboratory, for renovation, rehabilitation, rejuvenation, reintegration, resuscitation, etc." (Adams, 1985)

Osler's advice is as sound today as it was in 1905 when he addressed graduating medical students. Unfortunately, the intervening years have made it increasingly difficult to follow Osler's advice. The knowledge explosion of the latter half of the twentieth century increases the burden of keeping one's fund of knowledge current with each passing day. Much diagnostic and therapeutic information and technology are discovered every year. A common scenario at present involves the physician returning home tired each night to find one new major journal and three or four "throwaway" journals in the mail pile. He or she leafs through them (this takes a half-hour) and sees one or two articles in each that might be interesting. This adds up to five or six articles, too much for the already fatigued physician. He or she puts all the journals on the "to be read" pile. Over weeks to months, the pile grows, until it spreads over the physician's desk. At that point, in desperation, half of the journals are thrown out unread, while the other half are stacked on the shelf or bound (also unread). Too often, the surfeit of educational material overwhelms the physician and actually discourages him or her from reading any material.

How can the busy practitioner or the harried resident collect, savor, digest, and perhaps employ this new knowledge? The answer to this question is neither evident nor simple. Each new medical school graduate or experienced practitioner must answer this question for him- or herself. This chapter reviews the various postgraduate educational vehicles that are available and attempts to evaluate their usefulness and their role in continuing medical education.

Reading

Currently, there is an abundance of written material to assist physicians with continuing medical education: New textbooks appear with great regularity, older texts are constantly renewed, and a plethora of journals and monographs fills the mailbox of every physician. Some journals and monographs are published independently or by learned societies, while others are supplied by the pharmaceutical industry. Although material written by or for industrial sponsors may be accurate and educational, it is important to be sensitive to product bias as one reads these articles. A wealth of textbooks and monographs is produced each year. Many of these volumes cover similar material or represent collected papers from a congress or symposium. A brief examination of the table of contents and some spot reading will assist the physician in selecting the most desirable book.

Given the growth of medical knowledge, it seems wise to update those textbooks that are frequently employed (e.g., medicine, surgery, cardiology, obstetrics) with each new edition. Most students and practitioners will be best served by reading at least one general medical journal such as *The New England Journal of Medicine, The Lancet,* or *The Journal of the American Medical Association.* It is important to be aware of major medical advances in all fields. Subspecialists and generalists with a particular interest will want to read an additional one or more monthly subspecialty journals as well as occasional monographs. For example, one of these might contain articles reporting current research; the other might contain review articles. If time is short, one *must* guard against the tendency to read no journals because there are so many that one cannot possibly keep up. There is enough repetition in the literature so that all topics are eventually covered in each journal. Strive to read at least one journal faithfully.

Of course, the reader will not find every article in each journal to be useful or even intelligible. We have found the following system to be of value in reading medical periodicals. Read the abstract of each article. If it is something of interest, examine the article more closely: Read the introduction, examine the methods and results casually or intently (depending on interest), look at the figures, read the discussion for perspective.

In the course of reading an article, additional opportunities for education will arise. For example, concepts, laboratory studies, or etiologic theories that one does not understand well may be mentioned. It might take only a few minutes to look these up in a standard textbook. Older information is refreshed as one is acquiring new information, and the whole package is more likely to be retained. In addition, background articles of particular interest may be referenced in the article. This is another good way to broaden the educational impact. Finally, we believe retention is increased by topical reading when possible. One may want to cluster articles on a certain subject and read them at one sitting to increase the chance of retaining the new material, which is exactly what one does when preparing a lecture.

Any physician who has prepared a lecture or a conference on a particular topic recognizes the educational value of this exercise. During such preparation, the physician must master the material well enough to explain it clearly to others. Nothing surpasses this type of educational exercise with respect to retention of the material read. We, therefore, urge physicians to seek opportunities to give lectures or conferences. No one learns more than the presenter.

Finally, employ some method of recall. Some physicians rip interesting journal articles out and file them. This is an excellent system and can be highly recommended. We employ it ourselves. A word of caution: Save only very important articles lest the file becomes so large it intimidates its originator. It is also helpful to prune the file periodically when reviewing a topic or reading a related article. This allows the physician to eliminate less current articles while retaining more comprehensive or important communications. Some physicians prefer to prepare a file of reference cards for articles of interest. Some journals such as *The New England Journal of Medi-*

cine supply readers with such reference cards (they must be clipped from the magazine).

Recently, the advent of personal computers has led to a number of possible variations on these systems. The personal computer is employed as a file or is connected by telephone to a source of medical information and bibliography.

It is important that young physicians develop the habit of regular reading early in their careers. It is much more difficult to play "catch-up" than it is to keep one's education current by regular reading.

Continuing Education Courses

The years since 1960 have seen remarkable growth in quantity and, for the most part, quality of postgraduate medical education programs. These take a variety of formats: periodic lectures, conferences, or journal clubs organized by hospitals or groups of physicians; regional or national programs or courses involving lectures, demonstrations, luncheon panels, and discussion groups; combination vacation and educational programs that feature lectures and discussions during part of each of a series of days; intensive retreats usually featuring small group discussions; brief apprenticeships or short-review residency programs lasting for one to several weeks and usually available only at teaching hospitals; and audio or videotape presentations commonly offered at weekly or monthly intervals. Finally, the value of informal collegial relationships should not be underestimated as a tool for continuing medical education. Indeed, we have been impressed with the efficiency of this form of information-gathering, whether a quick question asked of a colleague in the halls of the hospital or a more official, formal consultation. Often, a brief telephone call to a knowledgeable colleague can solve a clinical problem or indicate that a more lengthy, formal consultation is indicated. Most physicians are flattered by receiving such a call; formal consultation can be requested if the situation turns out to be complex.

It is difficult to recommend any one of these learning programs as more valuable than the other. Individual physicians must experiment with different formats and then decide which is most valuable for them. We have been particularly impressed with the results of postgraduate apprenticeships or, as they are often called, mini-residencies. During such programs, practitioners return to the learning format that they employed during earlier internship and residency. During a period of one or more weeks (or one day per week for a number of months), the physician returns to a teaching hospital and participatcs in the daily educational experiences (e.g., rounds, conferences, lectures) of that institution. Suitable reading accompanies each day's work.

The Value of Continuing Medical Education

The amount of knowledge gained by individual physicians from various continuing medical education programs is difficult to quantify. A number of studies, employing a variety of test instruments, have shown that physicians fail to retain material taught in continuing medical education courses for more than a few days or weeks. Despite this lack of documentation of efficacy, most medical educators believe that some form of continuing professional education is essential for physicians. It is widely held that regular involvement in some type of educational activity prevents atrophy of the physician's overall knowledge. Physicians whose knowledge has become hopelessly outdated are not uncommon. In the absence of definitive evidence favoring one or another form of continuing medical education, each physician must create his or her own program of lifelong professional education. Most physicians find a combination program involving regular reading and attendance at some form of lecture program or mini-residency satisfies their needs.

Continuing Medical Educational Requirements

Many states require a specific number of hours of continuing medical education each year in order for a clinician to renew his or her license to practice. Recent trends have lessened the number of states requiring such professional education. However, as just noted, physicians who fail to renew their knowledge regularly find that their knowledge soon becomes outdated. Therefore, continuing medical education should be pursued regardless of local licensing requirements.

Suggested Reading

Adams, L. B., Jr. *Counsels and Ideals from the Writings of William Osler and Selected Aphorisms.* Birmingham: Gryphon, 1985. Pp. 172–175.

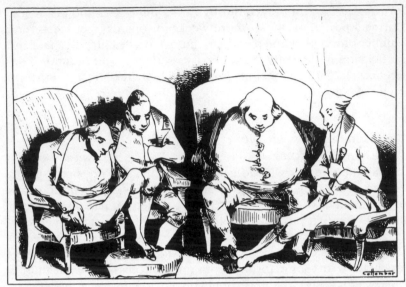

A satiric engraving depicting a group of gluttonous, soporific physicians holding a "consultation." (By the nineteenth-century French engraver Ratier.)

7. Role Models and Paternalism in the Physician-Patient Relationship

Patterning one's lifestyle or personality after that of another person is a common human response. At one time or another, we all employ this form of complimentary imitation. The advertising industry is based on this behavioral characteristic: The use of a particular product is tied to a popular sports figure or entertainment personality. The implication is clear: Use this product, and you too will look like, feel like, perform like the associated personality.

In the advertising industry, choosing a role model is a trivial but common example of behavior that is often employed by young physicians during the early phases of their career. Of course, role models can be used as a learning technique by physicians at any phase of their development. Medical schools consciously or unconsciously suggest role models for student physicians in the form of faculty members. In the recent past, a common medical school role model was the following: A dynamic, energetic physician who spent 10 to 11 months per year in a basic science laboratory (e.g., biophysics or biochemistry) and then emerged from the laboratory to dazzle medical students and residents with acute clinical acumen during a 1-month stint as an attending physician on the internal medicine service. The implications of such a role model were that (1) the ideal physician spent most of his or her time doing laboratory science, and (2) clinical medicine was a rather simple but nonetheless interesting hobby to be pursued for a brief period of time during the year. Changing social and professional conditions have resulted in a gradual change in the physician role model presented in most medical schools. The clinical investigator who dedicates a significant portion of his or her time to clinical medicine has emerged in the 1980s as the dominant role model in American medical schools. This change in medical school role models is a reflection, at least in part, of an alteration in career interests of many medical students. Few contemporary medical students seek a career in basic science; most are looking for a position with a heavy if not exclusive emphasis on clinical medicine. Thus, the Oslerian physician has reemerged as the dominant role model influencing current medical student professional behavior.

Sir William Osler was a Canadian-born and trained physician at the turn of the century who is largely responsible for the present American system of bedside clinical teaching. In fact, the term *rounds* originated at Johns Hopkins University School of Medicine during Osler's time there: The patient floor where he worked and taught was round. Thus, the word rounds was coined to describe his daily trip from bed to bed on that floor. Osler wrote extensively on the etiology, presentation, and management of illnesses that are dealt with by internists. He wrote a textbook of medicine that was considered the bible of internal medicine for several generations of American physicians. Moreover, Osler was a major force in establishing, during his lifetime, the preeminence of the Johns Hopkins University School of Medicine. Thus, Osler may be accurately described as the father of modern American medical education. He emphasized the importance of a careful and thorough history and physical examination as the first step in the analysis of the patient. The image of Osler teaching and investigating disease with the patient's bedside as the starting point has become the image for which many contemporary medical school clinical faculties strive.

This discussion is not meant to convince contemporary medical students that they must choose among different role models on the faculty in the same way that they explore different clinical disciplines in order to decide which postgraduate internship to select. Rather, these comments are offered in the hope that young physicians will become aware of the process of choosing a role model and will recognize this common human behavior. It is, of course, reasonable for a young physician to model his or her professional behavior after that of an older, admired colleague. Such behavior is not mandatory, however. In addition, slavish imitation is not conducive to normal professional growth and development. For many current physicians, choosing a role model means selecting a variety of different characteristics from different physician models. One might imitate the patience and tolerance of one physician and the energy and tireless work of another. Certain features will hopefully be common to all physician role models: compassion, empathy and kindness for the patient, dedication, industry, and honesty.

The Oslerian model—the astute clinician with keen bedside skills and a thoughtful understanding of pathophysiology—is a valuable legacy. However, there are other images in the medical heritage that are not so desirable. One such trait is *paternalism,* a behavioral trait that is best discarded by young physicians. Individuals who are sick often evince dependent behavior towards physicians and nurses. Such childlike behavior encourages paternalistic responses from health care professionals. The power given to the physician in the clinical setting often reinforces paternalistic behavioral traits. An example follows:

A 50-year-old man suffers an acute myocardial infarction. His hospital course is complicated by the development of ventricular arrhythmias and episodic left ventricular failure. Eventually, medical therapy suppresses these complications, and the patient is discharged to home to be followed as an outpatient by the cardiologist. During the hospitalization, the patient becomes extremely dependent on his physician and the nursing staff. He is now fearful of performing any activity without direct permission from the physician or nurse in attendance. His cardiologist fails to encourage independence on the patient's part and, in fact, states on several occasions that he "will take care of everything" and that he will "make sure things stay under control." Following discharge, the patient incessantly phones the physician's office with questions of minor importance. His postinfarction rehabilitation is markedly retarded by his dependence.

This cardiologist failed to encourage independent behavior from the patient. Consequently, the patient grew more and more dependent on the physician while the physician treated him as a child. The vicious cycle of patient dependence and physician paternalism had a strongly negative influence on the patient's convalescence. A more beneficial response on the part of the physician would have been to notice the patient's dependent behavior and carefully explain to the patient that the complications he was experiencing were very common in heart attack patients and would gradually subside. Finally, he might have expressed his confidence in the patient's ability to increase activity gradually toward a normal lifestyle with the assistance of the cardiac rehabilitation team.

In this manner, the physician would assist the patient in resuming a normal, independent lifestyle rather than continuing a passive, dependent existence. This latter scenario represents a superior role model for young physicians when compared to the initial response of the cardiologist.

Another issue relevant to the problem of paternalism is the manner in which a physician addresses the patient. It was common in an earlier era for physicians (then predominantly men) to address female patients by their first name. Moreover, it was also common for health care professionals to use terms of familiarity such as "dear" or "honey" when addressing patients, particularly women. These paternalistic forms of address are major sources of irritation to many people. Thus, "Mary, dear, would you please take a deep breath?" is inappropriate for current health care professionals. A more acceptable form of address would be, "Ms. Jones, would you please take a deep breath?" Of course, there are patients who prefer the physician to address them by their first names. It is reasonable to accept such patient requests and address patients thereafter by their first names.

Another form of paternalism occurs when the physician makes unilateral decisions for the patient without prior discussion or with only the most modest input from the patient. Many patients want to be involved in the selection of diagnostic and therapeutic options. Of course, patients look to their physicians to make sound recommendations concerning the advised course of action. However, patients are happiest when they participate in such decisions rather than merely accept the physician's paternalistic decision. The following example contrasts a paternalistic approach with a more egalitarian method of dealing with a serious problem:

M. J. has had a recent Pap smear that has demonstrated atypical, possibly malignant cells.

Paternalistic Physician: Well, M. dear, your Pap test wasn't completely normal, and so I'm going to perform a cervical biopsy. My nurse will help you prepare for the procedure.

Sensitive Physician: Ms. J., your Pap smear was modestly abnormal. I can't be sure, but it is possible that you have early premalignant changes in your cervix. I would like to perform a biopsy to see exactly what is going on. Do you have any questions?"

The paternalistic physician addresses the patient inappropriately and then tells her what he or she has decided to do. He or she fails to elicit the patient's feelings about the planned biopsy and fails to answer the numerous questions that undoubtedly assail the patient. The sensitive physician addresses the patient appropriately, explaining the clinical dilemma briefly and eliciting the patient's response. Further discussion will undoubtedly result. In the final analysis, the sensitive physician's patient is better prepared to undergo the biopsy and to accept the results. The sensitive physician and his or her patient are engaged in a diagnostic-therapeutic contract that will hopefully lead to a mutually satisfactory outcome. The paternalistic physician has enforced his or her will on the patient; the eventual outcome is likely to be far less satisfactory.

Suggested Reading

Coles, R. *William Carlos Williams—The Doctor Stories.* New York: New Directions, 1984.

Cushing, H. *The Life of William Osler.* Oxford, Engl.: Clarendon, 1925.

II. The Physician's Daily Routine

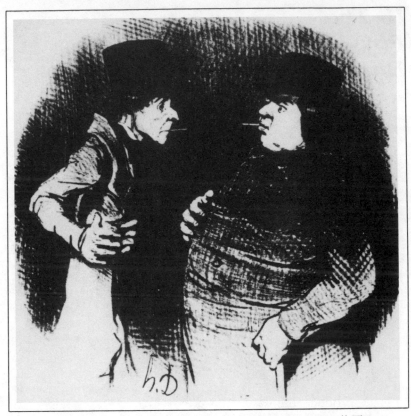

"Camphor Cigarettes." The conversation that accompanied this
lithograph read, *"I've been told
they're wonderful for putting on
weight!" "And I've been told
they're infallible for reducing!"
(Lithograph by Honoré Daumier,
1808–1879.)*

8. Wellness

Wellness is a term much abused recently by loose and overzealous application. Originated by the family health–holistic medicine movement, it was originally meant to imply a system of medical care that emphasized preventive medicine and a healthy lifestyle. In recent years, the definition of wellness has been broadened to include a vague series of so-called preventive medical measures such as a healthy diet, aerobic exercise, a yearly physical examination, and certain laboratory tests. The term itself has attained cliché status and is probably best forgotten. However, the concept that led to its original use is still useful and should be retained: an emphasis in daily clinical practice on those measures that should be incorporated into the lifestyles of citizens in order to minimize the risks of developing a variety of health conditions.

It is now generally agreed that the pathophysiologic sequences that lead to a variety of diseases consist of a series of interactions between the patient's genetic potential and specific environmental factors. For example, atherosclerotic coronary artery disease has a multifactorial origin. Hereditary factors such as blood pressure, cholesterol synthesis and metabolism, platelet adhesiveness, and vascular endothelial susceptibility combine with environmental influences such as cigarette smoking, diet, inactivity, and psychologic stress to produce the atherosclerotic lesion. Recent declines in coronary heart disease mortality in the United States are largely the result of recognition by physicians and the general public of the factors that lead to coronary atherosclerosis, with consequent attempts to reduce or eliminate risk factors from the lifestyles of large segments of the population. An example of such risk factor reduction follows:

A 35-year-old man seeks advice from his primary care physician. The patient comes from a family with a striking history of premature coronary atherosclerosis, with many first-degree relatives developing myocardial infarction or sudden cardiac death before the age of 50. The patient is asymptomatic, smokes one pack of cigarettes per day, is 20 pounds overweight, is sedentary, and has a serum cholesterol of 260 mg per dl. He loves to eat eggs, steak, and ice cream.

The physician counsels a gradual but significant change in lifestyle for this patient. Over the next 12 months, with the aid of the physician, a dietician, and a smoking cessation program, the patient stops smoking, loses 20 pounds, and changes his diet. He stops eating eggs, ice cream, rich cheeses, and red meats and markedly increases his intake of fruits, vegetables, cereals, pasta, and fish. He begins a progressive exercise program. One year after his initial visit, the physician and patient reassess the progress of the last 12 months. The patient is cigarette-free, he performs aerobic exercises for 30 minutes 5 days a week, and his serum cholesterol is now 190 mg per dl.

Both physician and patient are satisfied with the results of the preventive measures instituted. Moreover, the patient understands that his lifestyle changes do not guarantee that he will never develop the illness that has plagued his family. Rather, the patient's lifestyle changes reduce his *risk* of developing coronary heart disease.

A number of habits and environmental factors have been associated with an increased or decreased risk for the development of specific diseases. A brief discussion of some of these factors follows.

Factors Affecting Risk
HEALTH-PROMOTING FACTORS
EXERCISE. Regular exercise contributes significantly to the prevention of a number of clinical conditions including obesity, vascular disease, constipation, and certain psychologic complaints such as chronic insomnia. Excessive exercise can lead to musculoskeletal injuries such as tendonitis, bursitis, osteoarthritis, and even small stress fractures in bones in the lower extremities. A sense of well-being and even euphoria is commonly reported by individuals who exercise regularly, and this positive frame of mind has been attributed to increased central nervous system levels of endorphins generated by regular exercise. Conditioning programs have been employed with considerable success in the management of atherosclerotic coronary artery and peripheral vascular diseases and chronic obstructive pulmonary disease. It is prudent for physicians to advise regular exercise for all healthy individuals who seek to maintain their disease-free state.

DIET. It is a commonly held axiom that "we are what we eat." Sports trainers, entertainment personalities, and a number of self-proclaimed diet experts recommend one or another type of diet for attaining or maintaining optimal physical conditioning or state of health. Many of these claims are without any scientific basis whatsoever. On the other hand, careful epidemiologic studies performed during the last three decades offer a number of clues concerning the best diet for health maintenance.

Atherosclerotic vascular disease appears to be related to high levels of saturated fat and cholesterol in the diet. Food items that should be eaten in moderation include red meats, high-fat cheeses, whole milk, ice cream, eggs, and chocolate. The American Heart Association has endorsed a so-called prudent diet for all Americans that contains modest amounts of these foods with increased emphasis on consumption of fish, poultry, skim milk and other low-fat dairy products, margarine made from unsaturated oils, fruits, vegetables, cereals, and pasta.

Recently, a variety of malignancies have been associated with increased consumption of certain foodstuffs. Based on a number of public health studies, it seems reasonable for all Americans to moderate their intake of smoked, salt-cured, or nitrate-containing products, as well as foods containing artificial coloring and flavoring. In addition, the ideal diet for prevention of malignancy should emphasize decreased intake of fat, especially in red meat, and alcohol, as well as increased consumption of fruits, vegetables, cereals, and grains containing bran. Vegetables such as cabbage and brussel sprouts seem to be particularly beneficial. It is interesting to note the similarity of the atherosclerosis prevention diet and the malignancy prevention diet. Both emphasize decreased intake of red meat and saturated animal fats together with increased consumption of fruits, vegetables, cereals, and grains.

PSYCHOLOGIC HEALTH. Modern, technologic society presents individuals with a large number of psychologic stresses: high-speed travel with change in climate and time zone; job-related pressures; mobility; decreased family, community, and religious support; and the ever-present threat of nuclear annihilation. Given these stresses, it is not surprising that anxiety and other neuroses are widespread. Such psychologic distress can be just as disabling as serious physical ailments. In addition, most major organic illness is complicated by psychologic disturbances such as depression, anxiety, insomnia, and inappropriate denial. Adequate care for patients with organic illness must include attention to psychologic problems that accompany the organic illness.

A 45-year-old man develops unstable angina and is admitted to the coronary care unit. At first, he is inappropriately jovial, flirting with the nurses and denying the serious nature of his illness. Following cardiac catheterization and urgent coronary bypass surgery for triple-vessel coronary atherosclerotic disease, the patient becomes deeply depressed and cries easily. He is unable to sleep and frequently displays hostility towards the hospital staff. The cardiac rehabilitation team recognizes that such psychologic disturbances often complicate the course of patients with ischemic heart disease. Daily counseling sessions with the patient's physician and the rehabilitation therapist are instituted. The patient's illness is carefully explained to him, as is the universal nature of his psychologic distress. He is supported and reassured about his recovery and excellent prognosis. Gradually, psychologic equanimity and appropriate behavior return.

Apparently healthy individuals may also experience psychologic disturbances as a result of life stresses. The physician may recommend daily meditational sessions, exercise, or professional psychologic counseling depending on the severity of the patient's distress. Prescribing a mild tranquilizer such as diazepam (Valium) for a short period of time may aid patients who are experiencing acute anxiety symptoms resulting from a particularly stressful life situation (e.g., death of a family member).

Psychologic distress is a common, serious health problem. Physicians must be cognizant of and comfortable with the identification and management of such problems.

RISK FACTORS

CIGARETTE SMOKING. Cigarette smoking has been associated with a variety of diseases including atherosclerosis of coronary, cerebral, and peripheral arteries, a variety of cancers, chronic bronchitis, emphysema, and peptic ulcer disease. Risk for these conditions increases with increased cigarette consumption and falls following cessation of smoking. Pipe and cigar smoking seem to be associated with fewer risks than cigarette smoking, perhaps because the individual uses these forms of tabacco less frequently during the course of a day. In addition, few cigar and pipe smokers inhale the smoke to the degree that cigarette smokers do.

Patients with established atherosclerotic vascular disease have markedly increased complications if they continue to smoke cigarettes. It is, therefore, imperative that such individuals cease smoking completely.

ALCOHOL. Excess consumption of alcohol is associated with a number of disease entities: cirrhosis, a variety of malignancies, trauma, pancreatitis, cardiomyopathy, neuropathy, and several forms of central nervous system dysfunction among others. It has been estimated that close to 50 percent of emergency room visits in the United States are the result of excess alcohol consumption. Most individuals learn to use alcoholic beverages responsibly and moderately so that positive social effects are maximized and negative health influences are minimized. However, a minority of the population seem to be incapable of moderate alcohol consumption. These individuals function in an all-or-none mode with respect to alcohol intake. Clearly, total abstinence is the only rational route for such individuals to follow. Once alcohol-related illness develops, total abstinence is essential.

DRUG DEPENDENCE. Many Americans become dependent on legal or illicit drugs. Some individuals become physically dependent, while others develop psychologic dependence only. Legal drugs that patients can become dependent on include diazepam, chlordiazepoxide (Librium), barbiturates, and a variety of other tranquilizers, sleeping agents, and of course, narcotics. Dependence on these drugs is usually physical, and a severe withdrawal syndrome that may include seizures can develop with drug withdrawal. Illicit or street drugs can induce physical or psychologic need depending on the agent. Illegal drugs include heroin, various amphetamine derivatives, methylqualone (Quäälude), cocaine, hallucinogens such as LSD and mescaline, and marijuana. Heroin and amphetamines induce physical dependence; the other agents produce psychologic dependence.

Withdrawal syndromes including, on occasion, delirium tremens may accompany abstinence from specific legal or illicit drugs. Complex neurotic and even psychotic episodes can accompany withdrawal of drugs to which individuals have become psychologically dependent. In addition, illicit drug use has been associated with a variety of infections (e.g., endocarditis, abscesses) or immunologic complications (e.g., glomerulonephritis, pulmonary fibrosis, hepatitis).

OCCUPATIONAL HAZARDS. A large number of occupational hazards have been identified including carcinogenic chemicals, irritating and poisonous inhalants, and potential sources of traumatic injury. Permanent disability can arise from a variety of industrial hazards. An entire field of study, occupational medicine, focuses on job-related illness or injury and its prevention.

The Patient's
Sense of Control

Patients vary in their desire for autonomy in medical decisions that affect them. Some individuals seek a partnership with their physician: Medical decisions are openly and frankly discussed and negotiated. At the other end of the spectrum lies the patient who passively accepts the physician's plans for evaluation and therapy. Some physicians prefer the passive type of patient because this individual is nonthreatening and easily managed. However, such patients can lead the physician to commit the sin of paternalism with assumption of an excessively patronizing and controlling attitude toward all patients. Since physicians have considerable power over the patient's state of mind, it is important to resist developing this approach.

A 60-year-old woman is admitted to the hospital for evaluation of fatigue, anorexia, and weight loss. An extensive work-up reveals that the patient has lymphoma, and a therapeutic course of antitumor drugs and radiation is recommended. The patient's initial response to her physician is hostile when told of her diagnosis and planned therapy. She speaks of leaving the hospital and not seeking further medical attention. An empathetic nurse discovers that the patient objects strongly to what she perceives as her physician's patronizing attitude: The physician is unilaterally making decisions that will affect the rest of the patient's life. The nurse tells the physician of the conversation with the patient. Subsequently, the patient and physician have a frank and open discussion of the perceived patronizing attitude and the patient's therapeutic options. A management plan is negotiated that is accepted by both individuals.

Primary Care

The central role of the primary care physician in a patient's health care has recently been rediscovered. Patients discern the true nature of a medical problem infrequently since they are not trained to do so. Often a subspecialist's opinion is sought inappropriately; time and money are wasted. It makes the most sense for patients to initiate their search for evaluation and treatment of illness with a primary care physician. Often this physician can treat it without further evaluation. If the illness turns out to be puzzling or requires surgical or highly technical evaluation (e.g., cardiac catheterization), the patient can be referred by the primary care physician to the subspecialist. Reassurance and explanation of a medical problem come best from a physician with whom the patient is well acquainted: his or her own primary care physician. This does not mean that subspecialists (e.g., cardiologists or gastroenterologists) deliver only highly specialized care. All such subspecialists train initially in general internal medicine. In fact, many internal medicine subspecialists continue to devote 30 to 60 percent of their practice time to primary care. However, the medical care system functions at its best if both patient and physician understand who is delivering primary medical care: an internist, a family physician, or an internal medicine subspecialist with primary care interests.

Primary care physicians need to concern themselves with a wide variety of problems. Thus, they cannot focus as closely on the highly technical aspects of each problem as they would like. The primary care physician should try to understand the illness in relation to the patient's total health and call for consultation from a subspecialist to assist with highly technical aspects of care such as the performance of angiographic studies. Primary care physicians are the key in making sure that patients understand and follow the practices implied in the concept of wellness.

Suggested Reading

Benson, H. *The Relaxation Response.* New York: Morrow, 1975.

Katch, F. I., and McArdle, W. D. *Nutrition, Weight Control, and Exercise* (2nd ed.). Philadelphia: Lea & Febiger, 1983. Chapters 11, 12; pp. 239–268.

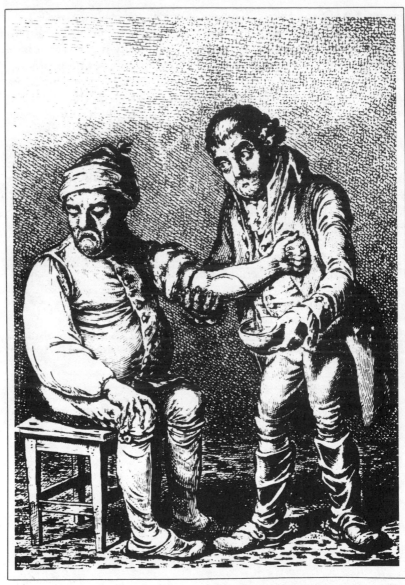

A physician bleeds a patient. The blood-letting is from an antecubital vein. (An 1804 engraving by James Gillray, 1757–1815.)

9. Treatment and Compliance

We preface this chapter on treatment by reaffirming what all physicians know: It is better to prevent an illness than to treat it. Yet treatment is much more dramatic than prevention and is, therefore, more often associated with the physician's role. We reaffirm another principle that physicians should follow: The best treatment is the least treatment that restores the patient's health. Treatment that can be accomplished without medications or surgical procedures is certainly the most desirable for the patient. Yet there is a mystique about pills, shots, and other physical treatments that compels patients to request them. Every practicing physician has repeatedly heard his or her patients ask, "Can't you prescribe something for this?"

Having stated our commitment to prevention and to physiologic rather than pharmacologic therapy, it must be acknowledged that an impressive array of treatments, including medications, radiation, and surgery, is available to today's physicians. The remainder of this chapter is devoted to a consideration of how these treatments can be delivered most effectively and humanely to the patient.

Form of Physician-Patient Interaction

It has been suggested that physician and patient can interact in five different ways during the treatment process.

1. Active-passive. In this kind of relationship, the physician is in complete control of the treatment. A good example is the treatment of a patient in diabetic coma.

2. Guidance-cooperation. In this interaction, the physician prescribes a treatment, but the patient must carry out the prescription. An example is 10 days of penicillin therapy for a streptococcal sore throat.

3. Mutual participation. This is generally an extension of the guidance-cooperation model. However, the patient plays a much larger role here. An example is an insulin-dependent diabetic who monitors urine sugar levels at home and adjusts both diet and insulin with periodic physician consultations and examinations.

4. Cooperation-guidance. In this kind of interaction, the patient designs her or his therapeutic regimen, and the physician provides help when appropriate. An example is a patient with mild hypertension who asks the physician to let him or her try a program of weight control, regular exercise, and relaxation techniques for blood pressure control, even though the physician is leaning toward therapy with medication. The physician decides to allow the patient to try her or his regimen and to cooperate in any way possible.

5. Passive-active. In this model, the patient demands and obtains a particular treatment. An example might involve a patient who calls up complaining of a bad cold and demands an antibiotic, which the physician gives her or him against the physician's better judgment.

The treatment model followed will vary not only for different patients but also for a given patient as she or he presents with different medical conditions and to different physicians. Some factors that will determine the particular model employed include the medical problem, the personality of the physician, the personality of the patient, and the physician's consciousness of the therapeutic process. It is this last factor, self-scrutiny by the physician, that we emphasize. Not infrequently, more than one model is possible in a given situation, and the physician must try to choose the one that is in the patient's best interest. An example follows:

A 42-year-old man consults a physician for hypertension. The patient has been to several physicians previously and has been very unhappy with them. He has been told repeatedly that his blood pressure is difficult to control. He has been tried on numerous medications, often with intolerable side effects. Inevitably, both he and the physician become frustrated and annoyed at one another, and the patient moves on to another physician. On this occasion, the patient presents with a blood pressure of 180/105 mm Hg, some arteriolar narrowing in the optic fundi, an otherwise negative physical examination, and photocopied records of a normal electrocardiogram, chest x ray, blood urea nitrogen, electrolytes, and intravenous pyelogram. He is taking a moderate dose of a beta-blocking drug once a day and nothing else. He has stopped his other medications, either due to side effects or mistrust of the physician. In particular, he fears hypokalemia, which has occurred on several occasions with diuretics and which once precipitated hospitalization due to abdominal cramps and a ventricular arrhythmia. During the visit, the patient is obviously nervous. Clearly, he is struggling with a mixture of fear about the blood pressure, dislike of medications, mistrust of physicians, and at this point, helplessness. The current physician decides to teach the patient to take his own blood pressure. The patient is skeptical at first, fearing that a high reading will upset him. The physician explains that blood pressures like 180/105 mm Hg will not harm the patient in the short term and that the patient's blood pressure will decrease with treatment. Most importantly, she tempts the patient with the idea of regaining control over his situation and no longer being completely at the whim of the physician. The physician also acknowledges the recurrent hypokalemia problem. She gives the patient larger than usual dosages of a potassium-sparing diuretic agent and sets up a schedule of frequent brief office visits to include determination of serum potassium. Over a period of 2 months, a regimen including high dosages of a once-a-day beta-blocking agent, moderate dosages of a thiazide diuretic, and high dosages of a potassium-sparing diuretic controls the blood pressure at levels below 150/90 mm Hg without major side effects. The patient takes his own blood pressure, which in the beginning is always lower at home than in the physician's office but later begins to correspond. The patient gradually becomes calmer, more trusting, and begins to feel well.

This patient was handled, as most patients with hypertension are initially handled, with a guidance-cooperation model. Early physicians prescribed a treatment regimen, and the patient was expected to cooperate. The last physician recognized that this model was not working. She realized that the patient needed more control over his own situation. Thus, she instituted a mutual participation model. This was more time-consuming for both physician and patient, but it worked where the other programs had failed. In most long-term illnesses, mutual participation or even cooperation-guidance model (i.e., allowing the patient to design the treatment to the greatest possible extent) works better than the more paternalistic guidance-cooperation model. Above all, the physician should be aware of what the interaction between her- or himself and the patient is, so that adjustments can be made if the treatment process is not going well.

Negotiation and Contract

Patients' expectations and physicians' recommendations are often in conflict. The disagreement usually stems from a different understanding of the medical problem or different expectations or preferences for treatment. When this occurs, it is the physician's responsiblity to explain the illness and then to negotiate a treatment plan that is acceptable to the patient and consistent with the physician's standards for good care. An example follows:

A 25-year-old woman presents to the physician with a severe sore throat. Examination reveals a temperature of 100.6°F, erythema and exudate on the posterior pharynx, and cervical lymphadenopathy. The patient has just begun a new job and wants medication to cure her quickly so that she does not lose time from work. When the physician suggests a throat culture, the patient objects, saying she does not have time to wait for the result.

Analysis of this seemingly simple situation is instructive. The patient and the physician are concentrating on different problems. The patient wants symptom relief since her primary concern is the ability to work. The physician is more interested in the etiology of the pharyngitis. He wants to be able to make a rational choice between antibiotic treatment to avoid the remote complications of streptococcal infection and symptomatic treatment to avoid a possible allergic reaction to antibiotics. If both the patient and the physician are to be satisfied with the outcome of this visit, some agreement must be reached. The interaction continues as follows:

The physician says, "It is obviously very important for you to feel better and minimize your absence from work. I will give you an anesthetic gargle, which will help. However, I would like to explain to you why the culture is important. . . ." He goes on to tell her about the possible consequences of beta-streptococcal infection and the reasons he prefers to give antibiotics only when *Streptococcus* is present. He also says, "Since time is so important to you, I could obtain the culture now and give you a small amount of penicillin to begin treatment immediately in case streptococcal infection is present. I'm going to ask you either to stop antibiotics if the culture is negative, or continue for a full 10 days if it is positive." The patient agrees to this plan.

In this scenario, the physician has determined the patient's primary concern: symptom relief. He has tried to deal with it by giving the patient an anesthetic gargle and conditionally prescribing an antibiotic. At the same time, he has explained his own concerns and negotiated a contract with the patient. He will begin antibiotic therapy now if the patient will allow the culture and stop the antibiotic if the culture is negative. The conditions for a successful contract have been met. Both parties are willing to negotiate. They have agreed on a plan. Each has responsibilities. Both stand to gain from the result.

Fitting the
Treatment to the Patient

In order to plan and communicate an effective treatment program, it is important for the physician to have some knowledge of the patient's intellectual ability, home and social support system, attitudes toward illness and different treatment modalities, general financial situation, and daily routine. Most of this information can be obtained during a standard history if the physician listens carefully. Sometimes specific questions are necessary to complete the picture. Examples of such questions include "Could you tell me your understanding of your problem?" "How do you feel about surgery for the problem?" "Is there someone at home who can help you with this treatment program?" "Will the cost of medication be a hardship for you?" "Is it possible for you to take medications several times each day?" Some of these considerations are illustrated in the following case.

A 76-year-old widower is referred to a cardiologist because of increasingly frequent chest pain. The patient has a list of medications that he is receiving. The list includes a digitalis preparation prescribed once per day, a diuretic prescribed twice per day, a moderate dosage of a beta-blocking drug, a moderate dosage of a long-acting nitrate, and a small dosage of a calcium channel blocking drug, all of which have been prescribed 4 times per day. When asked whether he takes all the medication faithfully, he answers, "I do the best I can." The cardiologist pursues this point, and the patient says, "The medicines are very expensive, especially the capsule [the calcium channel blocking agent], so I take that one twice instead of 4 times a day to make them last longer. Also, sometimes I forget which pill to take twice, and which 4 times a day." Further questioning about the chest pain reveals that the patient often has it after supper. "Since I live alone, many nights I eat supper at the diner on the corner. I get the pain while walking home."

Several features of this case are worth considering. The patient could not afford the medication as prescribed; thus, he decreased the dosage of the most expensive drug, negating its effect. In addition, he had a mild memory problem consistent with his age and no one at home to help. Therefore, he sometimes confused his medicines or forgot to take them. Finally, his life routine (i.e., having to eat out and walk home immediately after eating) facilitated his symptoms.

A fairly minor set of rearrangements, based on a knowledge of the patient's life routine and social situation, solved the problem. The calcium channel blocking drug, which he took only in low dosages, was stopped in favor of a higher dosage of nitrates prescribed in the generic form. This rearrangement markedly decreased the cost while increasing the efficacy. The physician had one of her office staff make the patient cards labeled "breakfast," "lunch," "supper," and "bedtime" with all the appropriate pills taped on each. This solved the memory problem. He was advised to wait a while after dinner before beginning the walk home or to take a prophylactic nitroglycerin before leaving the diner. This helped avoid the postprandial angina. This patient's symptoms improved on the new treatment plan. Control of the symptoms was possible only with knowledge of the patient's intellectual function, his home support system, his overall financial system, and his life routine.

Teaching

The word "doctor" is derived from the Latin *docere* (to teach). Indeed, in medical school and in residency programs, students and residents spend a good deal of time teaching one another. Yet almost no emphasis is placed on teaching patients, even though such teaching is the cornerstone of preventive medicine and a key component of therapeutic medicine.

The result is that physicians spend very little time teaching patients. One study found that physicians spent less than one minute out of a 20-minute visit communicating information about illness and treatment. Not only is the quantity of time spent small, but the quality of communication tends to be poor. Use of jargon is one of the many communication problems. A group of investigators compiled a list of 50 medical terms thought by practitioners to be appropriate for conversations with patients. The patients who were tested understood only a mean of 29 of these terms. Both the paucity of time spent and the impoverished level of communication contribute to the generally inadequate understanding patients exhibit when queried about their treatment programs. Another study demonstrated that 50 percent of patients could not state correctly how long they were to take medication. Moreover, 23 percent could not identify the purpose of the medicine, and 17 percent did not know how often to take it. To make matters worse, society in general seems to have accepted this situation. The *American Heritage Dictionary* has several definitions of the word doctor. Among them is *"obsolete. A learned person, teacher."* An example of such poor teaching follows:

A 55-year-old woman presents to a physician with a blood pressure of 170/100 mm Hg. After confirmation of the elevated pressure on another visit and some laboratory studies that suggest essential hypertension, treatment begins. The patient's pressure becomes normal after several medication increments at 1-week intervals. She is then scheduled to return every 3 months. Over the next 2 years, her blood pressure is in the 160/95 mm Hg range each time she is seen, and additional medications are added each time. Both patient and physician are frustrated. At one point, the patient goes to her employer and asks for a lower pressure assignment because her physician has told her she has hypertension. She is reassigned to a more menial, less satisfying job. The blood pressure continues to be elevated. In desperation, the patient switches physicians. The new physician, after close questioning, discovers that the patient omits her medication for approximately 1 day before each physician visit to see if her blood pressure has gotten better. In addition, she thinks her hypertension, which she understands as her level of stress, is causing her increased blood pressure. The new physician finally takes the time to explain that hypertension means high blood pressure, that generally it is a lifetime illness, and that medication must be continuous. After some teaching, the blood pressure is easily controlled.

This case illustrates the importance of being certain that the patient understands the illness as well as the treatment program. It also illustrates the pitfalls of jargon. The physician must leave time for explanations, must speak precisely but simply and omit medical jargon, must repeat, and must query the patient to ensure that she or he has understood. The query must be repeated on follow-up visits.

Compliance

A treatment regimen is effective only if it is adhered to. Unfortunately, noncompliance is a major problem. Multiple studies have suggested that noncompliance occurs 20 to 30 percent of the time when a regimen is curative such as an antibiotic for a specific infection, 30 to 40 percent of the time when the regimen is preventive, and 50 percent of the time initially when the treatment program involves a lifetime commitment.

The reasons for noncompliance are multiple and complex, and a detailed and scholarly presentation on the subject is given in other books (DiMatteo, 1982). We mention some of the more important factors leading to noncompliance in order to give the reader a basic understanding of the subject. The causes of noncompliance can be grouped under a few general categories. Some intellectual or psychologic reasons include failure to understand a physician's instructions, difficulty in remembering the instructions, psychologic denial of the medical problem by the patient, and regimens conflicting with peer group or cultural beliefs. Some environmental reasons for noncompliance include financial problems and time or scheduling constraints. Another very important cause of noncompliance is a poor physician-patient relationship. Some patients resist medical authority. They fear losing control over their lives. Instead of confronting the physician directly with this problem, they simply may not follow the recommended program. Other patients are intimidated by the physician. They may have cogent reasons for their noncompliance, such as side effects, but are afraid to report their problems lest they be judged ignorant or rejected by the physician.

The most important factor in maximizing compliance is good communication. The word "communication" comes from the Latin *communis* (common). The physician and the patient must have common goals, a common understanding of the medical problem, and a common plan for treating it. The cornerstone of good communication involves a clear and appropriate explanation. It is known that the more patients are told, the more they forget. Thus, a brief but relevant discussion may be best. Patients seem to remember best what they are told first and what they themselves consider most important. Thus, the instructions that the physician feels are the most essential should be mentioned early in the discussion and should be made relevant to what the patient feels is most important. The patient's educational background and general interests should be taken into consideration. Appropriate metaphors (e.g., subjects such as sports, automobiles, other hobbies) may be helpful in the discussion. After outlining a treatment regimen, it is important to elicit questions and objections, as well as particular problems that the patient anticipates. The physician should reinforce the patient's tendency to question or to voice concerns. Such statements as "That's a good question." or "I'm glad you told me that." will facilitate patient communication and thereby contribute to a mutually acceptable regimen. Finally, follow-up is essential. Patients must be asked during future visits how the treatment is going. They must be encouraged to relate problems rather than handle them with quiet noncompliance. A few points are illustrated in the following case:

A 45-year-old man has hypertension. The physician has decided to begin a beta-blocking drug. The physician has told the patient of the diagnosis and the preferred therapy. The physician might then say, "It is very important that you take the medication faithfully. We know that complications such as stroke can be avoided by good blood pressure control. It is also important for you to let me know if you have problems with the medication, so that we can alter it appropriately. Do you have any questions?" The patient might volunteer, "I have heard that blood pressure medicines cause impotence." The physician could answer, "I'm glad you brought that up. It is true that certain patients experience impotence with particular medications. Others have no trouble with the same treatment. If there is a problem, we can make changes, as long as you keep me informed. I am certain we can work out a program to control your blood pressure without disturbing your normal life routine."

In this example, the physician imparted to the patient the most important reason for compliance with medication. She or he has encouraged and then dealt sensitively with the patient's concerns. This type of interaction helps build rapport between patient and physician. It is crucial that physician and patient feel they are on the same team.

In summary, physicians must constantly remind themselves that it is better to prevent an illness than to treat it. If treatment is necessary, we must concede that the best treatment is the least or simplest regimen that will restore a patient's health. During treatment, we relate to patients in different ways. When possible, this relationship should aim toward mutual participation. We must not forget that physicians and patients often approach the same medical problem from a different perspective. The physician should try to attend first to the patient's concerns and then, if there is still a conflict, negotiate a contract that includes the physician's priorities. Teaching patients about their illnesses and their treatment programs is crucial. Ultimately, the degree to which the patient complies may depend on the patient's understanding of the problem and the solution, the degree to which the treatment program has been tailored to the patient's particular life circumstances, and the trust the patient has developed in her or his physician during the interaction.

Suggested Reading

DiMatteo, M. R., and DiNocola, D. D. *Achieving Patient Compliance: Psychology of the Medical Practitioner's Role.* Elmsford, N. Y.: Pergamon, 1982.

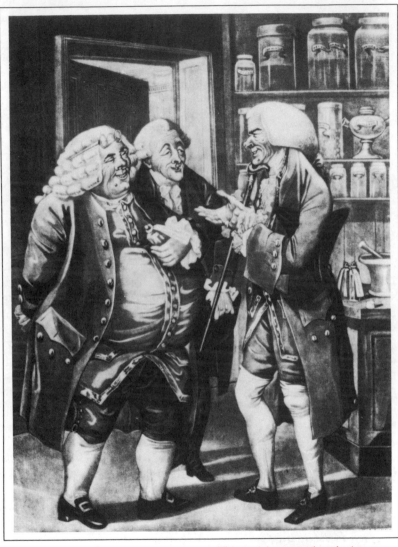

This satiric engraving depicts a consultation of pompous, self-satisfied eighteenth-century physicians. Under the engraving was the rhyme, "How merrily we live that doctors be, we humbug the public and pocket the fee." (By Robert Dighton, 1752–1814.)

10. Relationships

The practice of medicine requires the physician to be skilled in interpersonal relationships. These personal interactions take three forms: physician-patient, physician-physician, and physician-nurse. Successful management of most clinical problems demands that the physician maintain sensitivity with respect to these three areas.

Physician-Patient Relationships

One of the most important potentially therapeutic or harmful elements existing in clinical medicine is the personal relationship between physician and patient. Before the advent of effective medical and surgical interventions, the only positive therapeutic force that the physician could bring to the patient's bedside was a close, warm, and caring concern for the patient's life. With the advent of efficacious medical and surgical therapy, this positive force has been denigrated by some physicians who refer to it as "only a placebo effect."

It may well be that a positive physician-patient relationship involves factors resembling those called into play by administration of a placebo. However, such forces represent potentially powerful therapeutic factors, and as such, they should never be ignored or denigrated. Why not doubly benefit the patient with both efficacious medicine or surgery and the positive placebo effect (see Chap. 11) of a therapeutic interpersonal relationship.

Central nervous system (CNS) endorphin levels are apparently increased by certain positive interventions such as placebo administration. Endorphins have powerful CNS actions, and their presence in increased amounts following a positive placebo reaction is apparently of considerable benefit to patients with both minor and serious illnesses. Clearly, the clinician should accept all the help he or she can get. The therapeutic effect of a positive physician-patient relationship should *not* be ignored, even when effective medical-surgical therapy is available.

Patients listen with great care to everything the physician says. Frequently, patients misinterpret direct remarks from the physician or offhand comments made by one physician to another or by the physician to a nurse. It is, therefore, *essential* for the physician to choose words carefully when speaking to or in front of the patient. Physician behavior even in the vicinity of the patient (i.e., at the next patient's bed or at the door of the patient's room) may have an impact on the patient. The physician must draw on his or her empathetic powers, try to anticipate what words or behavior may be helpful or upsetting, and then attempt to act accordingly.

An overzealous but well-meaning surgical resident tells a recent vascular surgery patient that the latter's blood vessels were some of the worst that the resident has ever seen. The patient experiences a marked depression, and his postoperative recovery is long and arduous until the patient's family physician discovers the cause of the postoperative decline. A frank but reassuring conversation ensues; the patient's subsequent recovery is uneventful.

It has been said, somewhat tongue in cheek, that three essential qualities are required in a physician. In descending order of importance, they are

1. Affability
2. Availability
3. Ability

Although this triplet is meant to be sarcastic rather than realistic, there is more than a modicum of truth involved. However, the order of importance of these qualities is clearly inappropriate and should be

1. Ability
2. Affability
3. Availability

That a physician must be both intellectually and physically *able* goes almost without saying. A considerable fund of knowledge, good common sense, and a large store of stamina are prerequisites for most clinicians. Moreover, the clinician should be knowledgeable in social as well as basic science areas: A solid grasp of basic psychology, societal organization, and economics is important in daily clinical work. In fact, it has been suggested that the majority of patients seen in a primary care office setting suffer from psychosomatic illnesses, which are often the result of psychologic, social, and economic difficulties rather than organic factors.

Affability implies that the physician has a warm, friendly personality. Such qualities are reassuring to the average patient, who is often highly fearful of contact with the medical profession. Certainly, affability without ability often leads to deception: Quacks are usually affable but lack knowledge of medical science. Kindness rather than affability may be a preferable quality for physicians to cultivate. Patients are in an unenviable situation: They are usually fearful, uncomfortable, and weakened from their illness. Kindness in such a setting establishes a strong positive physician-patient rela tionship, often referred to as the *therapeutic partnership.*

The third quality appropriate for physicians is availability. The degree to which this characteristic is exercised is often cause for concern for physicians and their families. The nature of clinical medicine makes it a full-time job. Indeed, the more meticulous the care given to each individual patient, the greater the number of hours in each day devoted to patient care. Every physician is aware of friends or colleagues whose personal lives have been destroyed by constant, meticulous, but overzealous attention to patient care. Dedication to patients is an important quality in a physician. Nevertheless, each physician must decide for him- or herself the amount of time that will be dedicated to clinical practice in response to the demands of patient care. Clearly, availability is a two-edged sword.

Finally, it should be stressed that physicians need a certain amount of breathing room between themselves and their patients. This allows for objective evaluation of the patient's problems. An example follows of a physician who lost some of his objectivity and thereby served his patient poorly:

A 50-year-old physician is consulted by his brother because of an annoying tendency toward constipation, which has developed over the preceding 6 to 8 months. At least partly because he does not wish to consider a diagnosis of colonic malignancy in a loved one, the physician reassures his brother and gives him some sample pills of a stool-softener. The brother's constipation eases somewhat with this therapy but then returns. The patient, reassured that his brother seems unconcerned, ignores the increasingly difficult bowel movements, choosing to treat the constipation with patent medicines so as not to inconvenience his brother further. The two brothers are distraught when, 6 months later, the patient is diagnosed as having advanced cancer of the colon.

The patient was so close emotionally to the physician that the latter was unable to exercise his normally acute, objective clinical judgment. The result of this unfortunate series of events was distressing for both the patient and his physician brother. A response that the physician brother might have employed with more propitious results follows:

The physician brother gently reassures the brother that his constipation is probably nothing serious, but a careful evaluation should be performed to be completely certain that nothing is amiss. The physician makes an appointment for his brother with an internist friend for whom he has great respect.

In this alternate scenario, the physician brother recognizes and accepts his nonobjectivity, particularly as it relates to a family member. He, therefore, solicits the opinion of another physician who is not so intimately involved with the patient. Despite the fact that most physicians like to believe that they are dispassionate and objective with respect to their clinical judgment, it must be acknowledged that we are all prone to subjective forces. Value judgments, prejudices, likes, and dislikes all influence clinical judgment at some level. The most one can hope for is to be aware of subjective influences and to attempt to recognize when they are influencing the decision-making process.

Physician-Physician Relationships

In Hippocratic times, physicians were synonymous with healing priests, who did what they could to relieve the patient's suffering within the confines of the temple. The therapeutic partnership with the patient referred to earlier represented the only tool for healing that these early physicians had at their disposal. Hippocratic physicians were all men, and their work, as well as their approach to the patient, occurred in an atmosphere of secrecy. Today, more than 2000 years later, some of the atmosphere of this secret brotherhood still hovers about the medical profession: Physicians are reluctant to speak ill of each other or disagree openly with a colleague's management of a particular patient; patient confidences are kept secret except when discussing the patient with another physician; finally, physicians would like to believe that they are capable, without outside influence, of disciplining those physicians who stray ethically or legally beyond the limits of correct behavior.

Such collegial behavior has considerable merit. It supports each individual physician and allows him or her to seek counsel from a colleague without fear of exposure or ridicule. From medical collegiality has grown the tradition of postgraduate medical education: physicians training physicians as they themselves were trained. Consultation between one physician and another is an outgrowth of the collegial tradition. Unfortunately, there is also a negative aspect to this tradition: Some physicians maintain silence or look the other way when a colleague acts inappropriately or erroneously. Hopefully, an awareness of the source of such behavior will aid individual physicians in deciding what is appropriate and ethical under such circumstances.

A special kind of physician-physician interaction occurs when a physician becomes a patient. The situation can resemble the previous example, in which a physician cares for a close family member: All objectivity is lost. Similarly, when one physician cares for another, the process of identification may interfere with good common sense, and clinical judgment may be distorted. Again, the only defense in such situations is an awareness of the potential problem on the part of the treating physician. It goes without saying that a physician who cares for him- or herself is placed in an even more tenuous situation. Except for the most minor problem, it must be said that "the physician who cares for him- or herself has a fool for a patient."

In summary, the supportive aspects of physician collegiality provide the profession with one of its greatest strengths. Collegiality should not be abused in situations where common sense and ethical considerations dictate otherwise.

Physician-
Nurse Relationships

Physician-nurse relationships have been the focus of numerous novels, short stories, and films. Besides the obvious (and outdated) romantic implications of a largely male profession interacting with a largely female profession (the sexual representations of both groups have undergone significant changes in recent years), the physician-nurse relationship is often portrayed as a power struggle in the arena of clinical decision making. While both of these stereotypic relationships did or do exist, their incidence and importance have been exaggerated by television soap operas. In general, physician-nurse interactions usually occur at a high professional level, with each group having considerable respect for the other. Clinical medicine can be both exhausting and anxiety-provoking. Both physicians and nurses are prone to job-related depression and anxiety, often turning to each other for support. Moreover, the close working contact present between these two professions usually leads to collegiality with attendant educational and supportive benefits.

Problems arise in the physician-nurse relationship when physicians patronize or put down nurses, and when the latter attempt to assume extensive control of various aspects of patient management. The following two examples illustrate these problems:

A physician walks up to the revolving chart rack in the nurses' station. He begins to spin the rack to find his chart. As the rack begins to turn, he feels resistance, looks down, and sees that a nurse sitting at the table is just pulling a chart out as he begins his search. He gives her a quick glance, then proceeds with his search. The chart is not in the rack. He goes to the front desk and asks if anyone has X's chart. A nurse answers that he has it and is charting medicines. The physician walks over and picks up the chart from in front of him.

This physician does not understand that both he and his nursing staff are partners on the health care team. He should have apologized to the first nurse for not seeing her hand on the rack. He should have asked the second nurse whether he could have the chart when the nurse was finished.

A physician and a nurse are working together in a patient's room in the cardiac care unit. The nurse is giving intravenous propranolol in 1-mg increments as the physician monitors the blood pressure and heart rate. When the syringe with 5 mg of propranolol has been given, the physician asks the nurse to make up another 5 mg of the drug. The nurse leaves the room. After she has not returned 10 minutes later, the physician leaves to see what is taking so long. Someone else tells her that the nurse has gone to look up the maximum allowed dosage of intravenous propranolol. She has never given more than 5 mg of intravenous propranolol and is upset.

The nurse does not understand the physician's responsibility for the care of the patient. Instead of leaving and investigating behind the physician's back, she should have taken her aside, expressed her concern directly, and received a satisfactory answer, or politely asked her to administer the drug herself.

Physicians and nurses play crucial, complementary roles in patient care. Conflict between the two professions can only be detrimental to patient care. Such disagreements must be dealt with openly and with candor. Two facts must be kept in mind: Ultimate control of patient management is the responsibility of the physician, and nurses spend many hours each day with an individual patient while the physician sees the patient for only a few minutes. Observations made by nurses during these long periods of time are often of considerable assistance in planning diagnostic or therapeutic strategies. It is of considerable interest that experienced malpractice lawyers focus on the nurses' notes in the patient record as the most valid reflection of what was actually happening to the patient during a contested incident. Physicians should take the hint and read the nurses' notes as well as elicit their observations during rounds.

In summary, the physician-nurse relationship is one of the most important psychologic unions in clinical medicine. It is almost always a positive interaction that leads to coordinated care. Problems that arise between physicians and nurses should be dealt with as rapidly as possible since they can only lead to a compromise in patient care.

Suggested Reading

Ad Hoc Committee on Medical Ethics, American College of Physicians. American College of Physicians ethics manual. Part I: History of medical ethics, the physician and the patient, the physician's relationship to other physicians, the physician and society. *Ann. Intern. Med.* 101:129, 1984.

Weil, A. *Health and Healing—Understanding Conventional and Alternative Medicine.* Boston: Houghton Mifflin, 1983.

III. Specific Problems Encountered in the Practice of Medicine

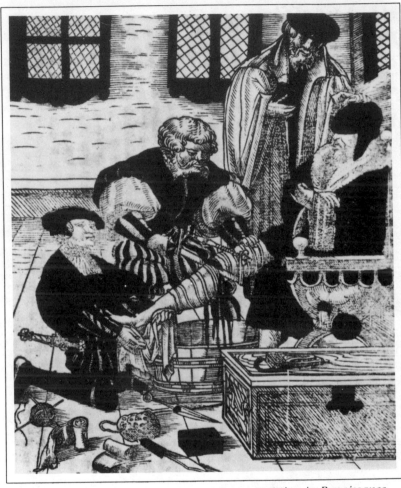

*An amputation in Renaissance
England. (From Thomas Gale,*
Certaine Works of Chirurgerie.
1559.)

11. Management of Pain

For thousands of years, physicians have been called upon to manage pain. No form of human suffering is more feared than pain. Therefore, it is not surprising that the practice of medicine often focuses on pain control. Analgesic (pain-relieving) drugs such as alcohol and opium and physical measures like acupuncture have been employed for centuries in the management of pain. Recently, a variety of newer pharmacologic agents and improved nerve-stimulating devices have enhanced the potential for pain control.

Before discussing strategies for pain management, a brief discussion of the physiology of pain is in order.

The sensation of pain is part of an important warning system that alerts the organism to tissue injury. Intense stimulus applied to living, innervated tissue leads to activation of nerve endings. Nerve impulses travel to the spinal cord where they activate a complex signaling system that can either relay these impulses to the cerebral cortex or suppress them. Certain local therapies such as acupuncture, massage, and electrical nerve stimulation activate a suppressor system within the spinal cord, thereby decreasing or abolishing pain. If the suppressor system in the spinal cord does not interfere with the peripheral nerve stimuli, then they are relayed to the brain and lead to recognition of the painful stimulus. However, a second pain-modulating (suppressing) system exists within the medulla and midbrain. Analgesia is produced by this system as a result of release of neurotransmitters, known as endorphins, within the central nervous system. These substances are actually endogenous opiates that suppress the perception of pain. Psychologic factors (e.g., anxiety) may play in an important role by preventing the activation of endorphin in pain suppression. Specific receptors on brain neurons are activated by endorphins or exogenously administered opiates (e.g., morphine), leading to analgesia.

Thus, patients with pain have at least two (and possibly more) endogenous systems for suppressing severe pain. A great deal of evidence points to activation of the brain-based endorphin system as the mechanism behind placebo pain relief. This accounts for the fact that psychologic factors involved in placebo administration are of considerable importance in determining the magnitude of the placebo response. In addition, the analgesic potency of a narcotic is

95

also tied to the psychologic state of the patient at the time the drug is administered. This means that placebos or narcotics administered with kindness and encouragement, as well as reassurance concerning their efficacy, will be more effective than the same agents given without psychologic support. Thus, it is imperative that physicians and other health care professionals employ supportive psychologic strategies in parallel with the administration of analgesic drugs.

A 47-year-old woman has been suffering from migraine headaches since her early twenties. She has seen a number of physicians (including specialists) who have examined her briefly and prescribed a variety of analgesic drugs. None of these physicians has ever carefully discussed her condition and its management with her. Finally, an experienced physician examines the patient carefully, explaining the etiology of migraine headaches, as well as the therapeutic strategies employed in their control. The physician's explanation emphasizes that migraine headaches are very common, that this problem frequently affects intelligent, motivated individuals, that migraine headaches are almost always benign and do not lead to strokes or brain tumors, and that therapy combining analgesic drugs and relaxation exercises often decreases or completely abolishes the headaches. The physician emphasizes his support for the patient and his desire to form a therapeutic partnership with her in order to control her migraine attacks. A combination of analgesic drugs and meditation exercises brings this patient's headaches under good control.

Analgesic Drugs

Pain sensation involves two types of neural systems: a transmission system for carrying nerve messages to the spinal cord and brain, and pain suppression systems in the spinal cord and brain capable of interfering with central nervous system perception of pain. Some analgesic drugs like aspirin, acetaminophen (Tylenol), and other so-called nonsteroidal antiinflammatory agents (e.g., ibuprofen [Motrin], indomethacin [Indocin], naproxen [Naprosyn], sulindac [Clinoril], fenoprofen [Nalfon]) block peripheral nerve transmission and thereby prevent nerve impulses from reaching the spinal cord and ultimately the brain. Opiates (e.g., morphine, meperidine [Demerol], methadone, codeine, pentazocine [Talwin]), on the other hand, owe their analgesic effect to their endorphinlike action within the central nervous system. These latter agents mimic the effect of the endogenous endorphin-mediated pain suppression system. Since antitransmission drugs and endorphinlike drugs act at different sites in the pain perception hierarchy, it is rational to combine smaller dosages of two agents, one from each category, in order to magnify analgesic efficacy.

Since opiates owe their efficacy to direct action on central nervous system neurons, direct injection of opiates into the epidural or intrathecal space produces potent analgesia. A small plastic cannula placed in this space can be utilized to administer morphine to patients with lower body pain (e.g., cancer or postoperative patients), for many weeks if required. Since smaller dosages of morphine can be employed, sleepiness and respiratory depression are less common than with intravenous administration of morphine.

Modification of neural transmission within the central nervous system by drugs other than narcotics can also produce analgesia. Serotonin is one of the most important neurotransmitters in the central nervous system. Drugs that affect serotonin metabolism and uptake (e.g., tricyclic antidepressants such as amitriptyline [Elavil]) can decrease pain in certain conditions such as migraine headache and postherpetic neuralgia.

Finally, it should be reemphasized that the placebo-induced activation of the endogenous endorphin pain suppression system should not be ignored. Physicians can use this response to the advantage of the patient even when effective pharmacologic agents are prescribed. Since such placebo relief of pain can be elicited in patients with intense physical discomfort (e.g., the pain of trauma or of malignancy), placebo response should never be taken as proof that patient discomfort is psychogenic in origin.

In general, physicians should try nonnarcotic analgesic drugs for pain relief before utilizing opiates. Even severe pain will often respond to aspirin or acetaminophen. Combination tablets of aspirin, acetaminophen, and codeine are highly effective analgesics for severe pain. Parenteral narcotics should be reserved for special circumstances such as acute myocardial infarction or postoperative pain.

Pain relief is one of the physician's greatest assets. No patient with legitimate pain should be made to suffer because of the physician's concern for the addiction potential of administered narcotics.

A 50-year-old man has extensive metastatic cancer. He is constantly in severe pain and is described by his physician as "a complainer and manipulator" who is constantly seeking narcotics. The patient changes physicians. His new doctor feels that the patient's pain is legitimate and allows the patient himself to regulate his narcotic dosage thus: The patient takes the narcotics every 2 hours on a regular schedule whether pain is felt or not. Once total or near total pain control is achieved, the patient attempts to increase *gradually* the time period between dosages until a limit is reached, or pain returns. Thereafter, the patient takes narcotics with sufficient frequency to prevent the development of pain. The patient becomes pain-free as well as less irritable with fewer complaints once his pain is relieved.

This example underscores one of the major tenets of chronic pain relief in cancer patients: Frequent dosages of an analgesic drug taken *before* discomfort is intense keep patients from experiencing agonizing pain and, with it, the attendant deterioration in sociability. No human being can interact with friends, family, or medical personnel when intense pain is present. The same principle can be applied to individuals with pain secondary to a chronic condition such as rheumatoid arthritis. Round-the-clock aspirin or another antiinflammatory drug is often necessary in order for such patients to lead reasonably normal existences.

Psychologic and Physical Analgesic Methods

A number of psychologic and physical methods can be utilized to control chronic pain. Often, these nonpharmacologic modalities are combined with analgesic drugs in relieving chronic pain. Such combination therapy often allows patients to use lower dosages of analgesic drugs, thereby minimizing drug-related side effects or addiction potential.

Psychologic interventions include behavior modification techniques and meditational exercises. A number of meditational or yoga programs have been successfully employed in controlling pain and anxiety. All such programs consist of breathing exercises, frequently combined with a variety of different postural exercises. Exercise and massage programs may also be beneficial. Transcutaneous electrical nerve stimulation and acupuncture appear to activate the pain suppressor system in the spinal cord and are therefore useful in patients with both acute and chronic pain syndromes. A last resort in the management of severe, chronic, and unrelenting pain is surgical interruption of peripheral sensory nerves or sensory tracts in the spinal cord.

Suggested Reading

Beaver, W. T. (ed.). Appropriate management of pain in primary care practice. *Am. J. Med.* 77:1, 1984.
Kabat-Zinn, J. An outpatient program in behavioral medicine for chronic pain patients based on the practice of mindfulness meditation: Theoreti-

cal considerations and preliminary results. *Gen. Hosp. Psychiatry* 4:33, 1982.

Kabat-Zinn, J., Lipworth, L., and Burney, R. The clinical use of mindfulness meditation for the self-regulation of chronic pain. *J. Behav. Med.* 8:163, 1985.

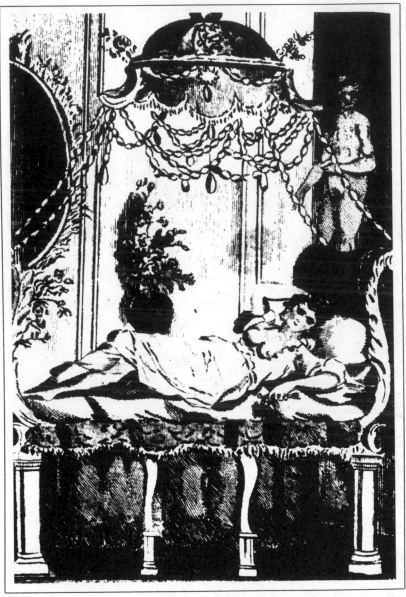

The Grand Celestial Bed of Health and Hymen, a device rented to gullible women by James Graham, an eighteenth-century quack. A childless woman could rent the bed for £50 per night in the hope of becoming fertile.

12. Management of Insomnia

Sleeps that knits up the raveled sleave of care,
The death of each day's life, sore labor's bath,
Balm of hurt minds, great nature's second course,
Chief nourisher in life's feast.

Macbeth

Physicians who take care of patients try to help them feel well. Patients who do not sleep well, do not feel well. Despite the fact that most healthy people sleep poorly some of the time and most ill people sleep poorly a great deal of the time, little taught in the classroom or the clinic enables the physician to be of help. This chapter outlines normal sleep patterns as well as provides basic information on the causes, effects, and treatment of insomnia.

Normal Sleep Physiology

The depth of sleep is described by stages, numbered from 1 to 4 with depth increasing as the numbers get larger. In stage 1, a person may feel wakeful, but studies in the sleep laboratory have shown decreased physical responsiveness and altered mentation. Stage 2 is the first true stage of sleep. Mentation during this stage consists only of broken fragments of thoughts. Stage 2 is interrupted by periods of rapid eye movement (REM) sleep, which occur in 90-minute cycles and last 5 to 15 minutes. Rapid eye movement sleep is complex, with some parts of the body relaxed (e.g., some striated muscles) and other parts of the body aroused (e.g., penile erections). Eighty percent of people who are awakened from REM sleep report dreams. Stages 3 and 4 (delta sleep) are the deepest stages of sleep.

In order to understand sleep physiology, one must look at it in two ways: the sequence of stages during a single night, and the changes in sleep patterns as one gets older. Several features of a single night's sleep are worthy of mention. The first is the delay from the time of going to bed until stage 2 sleep is reached. Both the latency period before stage 1 begins and stage 1 itself are experienced as wakefulness. It is a combination of latency and stage 1 sleep that most of us experience when we "lie awake for hours." Most chronic insomnia involves prolonged latency before falling asleep or persistence of stage 1 sleep. Once true sleep occurs, stage 4 (delta, or deep, sleep) occurs during the first 2.5 hours and is experienced as profound sleep from which one is awakened only with great difficulty. The remainder of the night is made up predominantly of stage 2 sleep, interrupted by REM periods and brief awakenings. Rapid eye movement periods occur with increasing frequency and intensity during the early morning hours.

Fig. 12-1. Development of sleep periods over a lifetime. The width of the various zones represents the amount of time spent in each of those sleep stages during a typical night by an average individual at different ages.

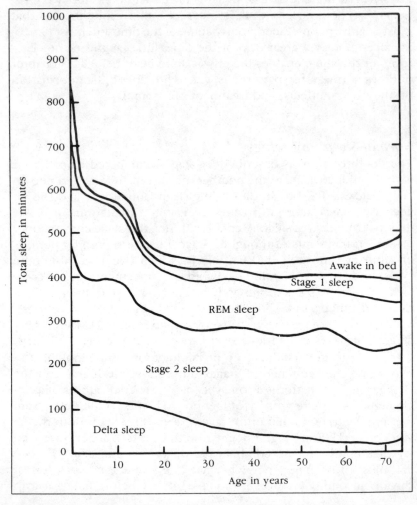

There are distinct changes in the pattern of sleep as one gets older (Fig. 12-1). The most obvious change involves the duration of sleep. As people age, they tend to sleep less. The change from infancy to adolescence is dramatic and from adolescence to old age more gradual (Table 12-1). Latency before falling asleep does not change with age. Instead, there is progressively less stage 4 sleep and more and longer awakenings during the night. Interestingly, total sleep time decreases until about age 59 and then increases again, mainly due to the addition of daytime naps. Older people, although they spend the same amount of time in bed at night, spend less of this time sleeping. They often find this change disturbing, especially if they do not know that it is normal.

Sleep Deprivation
Young, healthy volunteers do not have significant deficits in next-day performance after sleeplessness. They may notice a change in mood with increased irritability, or they may notice a decrease in vigilance. It may be more difficult to perform either very monotonous or creative tasks. Even after 2 to 3 nights of sleep deprivation, performance is not substantially affected, although microsleeps intrude into wakefulness. After several sleepless nights, 2 to 3 good nights of sleep will correct both the subjective discomfort and the sleep pattern.

Prevalence of Insomnia
Surveys (Kales, 1984) demonstrate that approximately one-third of people report difficulty sleeping at least sometimes. The prevalence of sleep disturbances is increased among women, older people, and lower socioeconomic groups. When asked, most people believe that they should obtain 8 hours of sleep. Yet only 20 to 30 percent actually attain this goal. Severe chronic sleep deprivation (< 4 hours/night) has been correlated with an increased mortality from heart disease, cancer, and stroke.

Table 12-1. Changes in sleep duration with age

Age (yr)	Duration of sleep (hr)
0–4	17–18
4–10	10–12
> 10	7.5, decreasing to 6.5

Causes of Insomnia

The situations that lead to disturbed sleep range from simple situational changes to complex medical problems. An example of a simple situational cause is jet lag, when a person's time clock is thrown off transiently. Jet lag can be minimized by beginning a trip rested. Other simple perturbers of sleep are unfamiliar environments (e.g., a hotel room or the hospital), markedly increased environmental temperature (above 75 °F), intermittent background noise, and central nervous system stimulants such as coffee, nicotine, and alcohol. Although alcohol may help one to fall asleep, it causes more frequent awakenings during sleep. Weight loss or hunger may disturb sleep. A snack before bedtime, perhaps even the old folk remedy of warmed milk, can be helpful. Poor sleep habits, including such things as frequent daytime naps, irregular bedtime, exercise, or upsetting activities immediately before retiring, can all disturb sleep.

Medical conditions that interfere with sleep are more complex but are often amenable to treatment. Some examples include peptic ulcer pain, nocturnal angina pectoris, and severe arthritic conditions. These are amenable to specific (or analgesic) treatment. Psychiatric conditions are very frequently accompanied by sleep disturbances. Anxiety syndromes generally affect falling asleep, whereas depression is accompanied by early awakening.

Iatrogenic causes of sleep disturbance are prevalent and sometimes preventable. A number of drugs may cause insomnia. Naso- and bronchodilators may cause symptoms due to adrenergic stimulation. Beta blockers are known to cause nightmares in some people. Diuretics may produce the frequent need to arise and urinate. Short half-time diazepines such as triazolam (Halcion) may cause rebound insomnia toward morning, especially if used for many days in a row. Anxiety in hospitalized patients frequently leads to insomnia. It is known that surgical patients sleep poorly before a procedure and that the severity of the sleep disturbance increases with the seriousness of the contemplated operation. When possible, adequate antianxiety or sleep medication should be prescribed. Sleep is interrupted even more dramatically in the postoperative state: Studies have shown more than 50 interruptions on the first night after a cardiac surgical procedure and more than five interruptions on the eighth night after such operations. The delirium sometimes seen in intensive care patients may, in part, be due to insomnia produced in this way.

An iatrogenic cause of sleep disturbances, both common and preventable, involves vital signs and physician-prescribed drug schedules. An example follows:

A 72-year-old man is hospitalized for unstable angina pectoris. He is first monitored in the cardiac care unit, and when a myocardial infarction has been excluded and the pain has been abolished with medication, he is sent to an adjoining telemetry floor. Each morning, his physician asks him how he is doing. Each morning, the patient gives the same answer. "I'm not having any pain, Doc, but I'm exhausted. I don't feel like doing anything." At first, the physician reassures the patient that the stress of hospitalization and the anxiety of the cardiac care unit have caused his fatigue and that he will soon feel better. However, the fatigue remains, and both physician and patient become frustrated. One day as the physician is leaving the room, the patient says, "Oh by the way, Doc, do I absolutely need that 4 A.M. medication?" The physician tells the patient that she will check the medication schedule and try to alter it. When the physician looks carefully at the medication sheet, it reads

Nitroglycerin ointment, 1 inch—12, 4, 8, 12
Propranolol, 40 mg—12, 6, 12, 6

The physician then realizes that the patient probably goes to bed at 11 P.M. and that his night is being interrupted at 12 A.M., 4 A.M., and 6 A.M. Furthermore, medication is being given during the day at 8 A.M., 12 P.M., 4 P.M., 6 P.M., and 8 P.M.—a schedule impossible to maintain after leaving the hospital. The physician goes back, speaks with the patient, and finds out that in addition to 12 A.M., 4 A.M., and 6 A.M. medication, blood pressures are sometimes taken at odd times like 1 A.M. On one occasion, the patient was awakened to see if he wanted a sleeping medication.

This case illustrates the importance of looking carefully at the times when medications are given. With the exception of very unstable situations, medication need not be given at exactly spaced intervals. Only rarely does it need to be given during the night. Angina pectoris is a good example. After stabilization in a cardiac care unit, dosages of medications are usually high enough to allow the night to be free of disturbance. Most medications can be given at or around mealtimes and at a reasonable bedtime like 11 P.M. Occasionally, a higher dosage is given at bedtime to carry the patient through the night. It may even be wise to write in the chart, *"Do not awaken the patient between 11 P.M. and 6 A.M. for vital signs or medication."*

Another problem hospitalized patients often face is a noisy roommate. The noise may be due to a medical problem that is accompanied by such things as loud respirations or expressions of pain. It may be due to frequent visits by the nursing staff. It may be because of personal habits such as watching late-night television. The physician must be alert to such things and rearrange roommates when appropriate.

Treatment

Treatment for insomnia will obviously vary a great deal, depending on the cause. As discussed previously, in-hospital causes of sleep disturbance may be relatively easy to identify and rectify *if* the physician is alert to them. Some of the time, hypnotic medications will be necessary in addition to the previously discussed strategies.

A detailed discussion of the pharmacology of hypnotics is beyond the scope of this book. However, a few principles of therapeutics may go a long way. Currently, the most popular hypnotics are the benzodiazepines, specifically flurazepam (Dalmane), temazepam (Restoril), and triazolam (Halcion). When prescribing a diazepine for sleep, one must consider certain questions: How quickly does it induce sleep? How long do the effects of a single dosage last? Does the medication continue to be effective with prolonged use? What are the side effects? Table 12-2 summarizes some of the answers to these questions.

Several points need to emphasized. Triazolam and temazepam have some advantages in older people because their half-lives are shorter, and thus accumulation over a few days with resultant daytime sleepiness is less of a problem. They are poor choices if a hypnotic must be given every night for more than a few days. They tend to lose their effectiveness after several days and, like other diazepines with short half-lives, cause early morning insomnia or, after stopping the drug, rebound insomnia. Flurazepam must be used cautiously in older people because of its long half-life. However, in a middle-aged or younger population, flurazepam offers advantages. It increases its effectiveness over the first 2 to 3 days, and it does not lose its effectiveness over time. It does not cause early morning insomnia. After discontinuation of the drug, the long half-life probably contributes to the absence of rebound insomnia. In addition, it causes rapid induction of sleep, a valuable property since most chronic insomnia involves difficulty in falling asleep.

Treatment of insomnia in outpatients should involve multiple modalities. First, it is important to define the sleep disturbance. Spouses should be queried when possible, as well as the patient. A

Table 12-2. Sleep medications: prescription information

Drug	Dose	Sleep induction	Half-life	Side effects	Effect with continued administration
Flurazepam (Dalmane)	15–30 mg	Rapid	50–100 hr	Daytime sleepiness	Good
Temazepam (Restoril)	15–30 mg	Slow	15 hr	Morning sleepiness; rebound insomnia	Poor
Triazolam (Halcion)	0.125–0.500 mg	Slow	2–4 hr	Amnesia; early morning insomnia; daytime anxiety; daytime sleepiness	Fair

history of excessive daytime sleeping, loud snoring at night, and periods of apnea may give the physician a clue to sleep apnea. In all patients, the pattern of the disturbance and the patient's manner of handling it should be explored. Is the problem one of falling asleep? Psychologic stresses or poor prebed habits can cause this. Is the problem one of staying asleep? Environmental problems, inappropriate drug dosing, and medical problems can all contribute. Is the problem one of early awakening? Depression often leads to early awakening, and antidepressant drugs with hypnotic properties, given at bedtime, may be helpful. Once the problem is defined, the treatment usually involves instruction for altering the sleep-wake pattern, psychologic counseling, and medication. An example follows:

A 54-year-old man who retired because of significant heart disease reports an inability to sleep. The physician questions him about the exact pattern of the disturbance. He answers, "I usually go to bed about midnight, I try to sleep, but I toss and turn and look at the clock, and sometimes it will be 3 A.M. or 4 A.M. before I fall asleep. I hate lying there in bed at night in the dark." The physician asks him whether he sleeps late in the morning. "Yes, I sleep until 10 or 11 o'clock." The physician questions the patient about when the sleep disturbance began. He says, "You see, I'm in the process of a divorce. My problem began about a month ago when the negotiations with lawyers began."

This situation illustrates a very common sequence in sleep disturbances. The problem began with the psychologic stress of a divorce proceeding. This stress is ongoing. Repeated insomnia at bedtime became self-perpetuating for several reasons in addition to the stress. The patient tried too hard to sleep, became frustrated and more aroused, and thus insomnia worsened. In fact, the patient admitted to dreading his bedroom. This association of the bedroom with insomnia is called *conditioned wakefulness*. Finally the patient began to oversleep in the morning, which changed his biologic clock and further perpetuated insomnia at his usual retiring time.

A suggested treatment plan illustrates several common principles of therapy. The patient was to have some counseling, either with his own physician or with a mental health professional. Clearly, some of the psychologic problems stemming from the divorce needed attention.

The patient is given a hypnotic (flurazepam, 30 mg) because it induces sleep quickly. The agreement with his physician is that he will use the sedative for 3 to 4 nights to break the cycle and then will have the sedative available but will not use it more than every third night. The physician instructs the patient to arise at 8 A.M. every morning, no matter how badly he sleeps, and not to nap during the day. This is intended to return the patient's sleep cycle to normal. Finally, the patient is told not to lie in bed for long periods awake. He is to get up, do something like read or watch television in another room no matter what the hour, and go to bed only when very sleepy. The bedroom needs to be reassociated with sleep, not wakefulness.

This case study is presented to illustrate the fact that insomnia often begins with some stressful situation, then becomes self-perpetuating due to fear of insomnia, conditioned negative responses to the bedroom, and resetting of the biologic clock. Clearly, the approach to complex problems such as this should be multidimensional.

The elderly patient deserves special mention. Several factors often compound to produce insomnia. As mentioned before, older people tend to sleep a shorter period of time, and their sleep is broken by more awakenings. It is important to explain to them that this is normal. In addition, they tend to nap during the day. This can be pointed out to them and accepted as part of the total sleep package or discouraged if they insist on a longer period in bed at night. Finally, older people have many objective worries and aggravations. These include loneliness, monetary difficulties, medical problems, and cognitive problems. Sometimes all of these problems must be considered when constructing a treatment plan. In the hospital, older people may become confused at night, the so-called sundown syndrome. It helps to leave a light on near them, and small dosages of haloperidol (Haldol), 0.5 to 1.0 mg, may be useful.

In summary, physicians need to understand and try to alleviate sleep disturbances. The complaint that "I'm having trouble sleeping" seems petty next to "I'm short of breath." or "I have squeezing chest pain." However, it is not petty in terms of *quality of life*. Most physicians are quite good at evaluating and treating shortness of breath, chest pain, and other tangible and dramatic problems. Most physicians are not skilled at handling insomnia and, thus, choose either not to hear the complaint or to prescribe a hypnotic summarily. This is wrong. It can be surprisingly satisfying for physician and patient when sleep disturbances are handled with interest, patience, and, after some practice, skill.

Suggested Reading

Hauri, P. *The Sleep Disorders*. Kalamazoo, Mich.: Upjohn, 1982.

Kales, A., and Kales, J. D. *Evaluation and Treatment of Insomnia*. New York: Oxford, 1984.

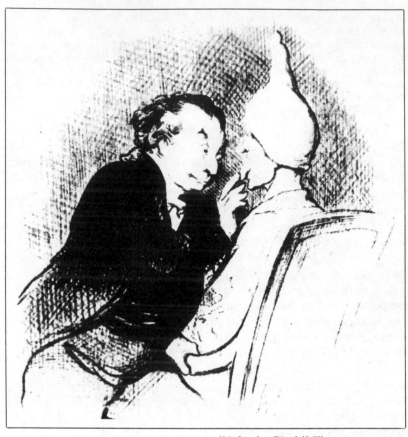

"A Lucky Find." The conversation that accompanied this lithograph read, "By Jove, I'm delighted! You have yellow fever. . . . It will be the first time I've been lucky enough to treat this disease." (Lithograph by Honoré Daumier, 1808–1879.)

13. Management of Fear and Anxiety

He remembered his medicine, raised himself, took it, then lay on his back observing what a beneficial effect the medicine was having, how it was killing the pain. "Only I must take it regularly and avoid anything that could have a bad effect on me. I feel somewhat better already, much better." He began probing his side—it was not painful to the touch. "I really can't feel anything there, it's much better already." He put out the candle and lay on his side—his caecum was improving, absorbing. Suddenly he felt the old, familiar, dull, gnawing pain—quiet, serious, insistent. The same familiar bad taste in his mouth. His heart sank, he felt dazed. "My God, my God!" he muttered. "Again and again, and it will never end." And suddenly he saw things in an entirely different light. "A caecum! A kidney!" he exclaimed inwardly. "It's not a question of a caecum or a kidney, but of life and . . . death. Yes, life was there and now it's going, going, and I can't hold on to it. Yes. Why deceive myself? Isn't it clear to everyone but me that I'm dying, that it's only a question of weeks, days—perhaps minutes? Before there was light, now there is darkness. Before I was here, now I am going there. Where?" He broke out in a cold sweat, his breathing died down. All he could hear was the beating of his heart.

Tolstoy
The Death of Ivan Ilyich

Patients know that illness is accompanied by pain, loss of normal function, loss of control, and death. This knowledge leads to fear (an emotional response to specific dangers) and anxiety (a similar emotional response but in the absence of a well-identified threat). At times, fear or anxiety may be so severe that it is the patient's most important problem. Physicians must learn to anticipate, recognize, and where possible, prevent or lessen fear and anxiety. This chapter presents some information on fear and anxiety and, more important, tries to stimulate the physician to be more sensitive to this problem.

Physical Manifestations

The physical manifestations of fear and anxiety reflect the intense autonomic activity that accompanies these emotions. In Martha Weinman Lear's book *Heart Sounds* (New York: Simon and Schuster, 1980), she describes her physician husband's reactions during a cardiac catheterization:

"He looked up at the screen. There he was live on TV. He saw his pelvis, his bones, his spinal column. And then, in a corner of the screen he saw this thing, this intrusion, this snakelike tube beginning to creep into his pelvis. He was sweating harder. His body was rigid. His heart was pounding. . . ." (P. 115)

In addition to perspiration, tense muscles, and rapid heart beat, fear and anxiety can produce dry mouth, rapid breathing, faintness, paresthesias, a lump in the throat, and intensified consciousness of pain. This constellation of symptoms appears to reflect a general increase in bodily sensitivity and responsiveness. As part of the "fight and flight" response, these symptoms may be markers of the body's preparation for action. When no action is possible, they become very unpleasant sensations.

Physiology of Anxiety-Related Symptoms

In order to try and understand the physiology and biochemistry of the symptoms accompanying fear and anxiety, scientists have turned to very simple animals such as the marine snail *Aplysia*. Facsimiles of both anticipatory and chronic anxiety have been produced in this animal model.

The experiments are designed as follows: *Aplysia* responds to a weak tail shock with escape locomotion. An exaggerated response to the shock is used as a measure of anxiety in these animals. *Aplysia* has sensors that detect the presence of shrimp juice in the environment. If the animal receives a strong head shock each time it is exposed to shrimp juice, a behavior resembling anticipatory anxiety results. Exposure to shrimp juice followed by the weak tail shock causes much more vigorous escape locomotion than a weak tail shock in the absence of the shrimp juice (i.e., shrimp juice causes anticipatory anxiety). If, on the other hand, the animal is given strong head shocks without a warning stimulus such as shrimp juice, the animal, after a time, begins to exhibit a behavior resembling chronic anxiety. Any weak tail shock, no matter when given, whether with or without shrimp juice, results in escape locomotion that is more vigorous than if the snail had not been given the periodic head shocks. The animal has become chronically hyperreactive. *Aplysia* has a simple nervous system; these responses have been traced to neurons that release a serotoninlike substance. The serotoninlike substance stimulates adenylate cyclase, increasing the amount of intraneuronal cyclic AMP, thereby leading to phosphorylation of one specific protein. These anxious animals have persistent morphologic changes of their neurons, thereby presenting anatomic as well as behavioral and biochemical evidence of their learned reaction.

Work such as this suggests that the mind-body gap can be bridged and that we will eventually be able to deal with problems such as anxiety in a specific biochemical as well as the traditional interpersonal fashion. For the present, however, psychologic considerations remain paramount.

Psychologic
Manifestations of Anxiety

There are many psychologic manifestations of fear and anxiety. Some are more easily recognized than others. The patient whose handshake is cool and moist, who shifts position continually in her or his chair, or who makes frequent mistakes while speaking is sending out continuous signals of her or his anxiety. However, other patients who seem unconcerned or unimpressed or who appear to be very negative (sometimes even belligerent) may also be revealing their anxiety. It is important to recognize fear or anxiety whatever its guise and to try to lessen it. In the following examples, these points will be illustrated.

The first case concentrates on the management of overt fear.

A 65-year-old man is hospitalized because of chest pain. He has been a diabetic for 15 years and has required insulin for 5 years. The patient has always been nervous about his illness and has finally decided to resolve the situation with cardiac surgery. Coronary angiography reveals poor left ventricular function with an ejection fraction of 24 percent and severe triple vessel disease with enough distal vessel involvement to prevent effective coronary surgery. When the physician comes into the room to tell the patient the results of the angiogram, the patient is on the telephone. He sees the physician, abruptly interrupts his conversation, and says into the telephone, "I'll call you later. My doctor's here." He sits up quickly. His neck muscles are tense. His eyes are riveted to the physician's eyes. "I've been waiting for you, doc. How bad is it? Can surgery handle it?"

This patient's fear is obvious. The question is, how should the physician handle it? There is no single correct formula. The physician should close the door or curtain and sit down. She or he might say, "Mr. D., we obtained very good pictures, and I think they will be of great help in treating you properly. They suggest to me that it would be better to adjust your medications than to proceed to surgery. I know you were hoping for surgery, but sometimes the risks outweigh the benefits of the procedure. I think if we work together and adjust your medication, we can make you feel quite a bit better.''

Certain aspects of the physician's behavior are worthy of note. She or he sat down in order to reassure the patient that they were going to devote some time to the problem. The physician was honest, but the statement was positive, suggesting that action could and would be taken. The physician also implied that she or he would continue to help the patient. This type of situational anxiety is best handled by giving the patient time, showing that one cares and will continue to work on the patient's behalf, and emphasizing the positives—what *can* be done—while remaining truthful. The patient is apt to emerge feeling less anxious and sensing that she or he has a caring and powerful ally.

It would have served little purpose to say, "I'm sorry, I found your heart to be quite weak and your arteries too diseased to correct by surgery.'' Shakespeare, in *The Tempest*, commented on this approach:

"The truth you speak doth lack some gentleness,
And time to speak it in: you rub the sore
When you should bring the plaster.'' (II, i)

The next case presents an encounter with a patient whose anxiety is masked.

A businesswoman of 55 is found to have a lump in her breast on a routine examination. A mammogram suggests tumor. The physician advises her to have a biopsy and explains that the microscopic examination will determine whether or not she needs further treatment. The patient says, "This is a very busy time for me. I will call you in a few months to discuss it further.'' The physician responds, "I don't think you should wait. If it is a tumor, time may be very important in the chance for a cure.'' She says, "After I return from a business trip, I'll discuss it with my husband and let you know.''

It is quite likely that this patient is covering up her fear with denial. The physician, in an attempt to convince her to act, must keep the fear in mind and try not to worsen it. One way to do this is to allow the patient as much control as possible and to accentuate positive action. The physician might say, "I realize that you have a great many responsibilities. Surely, one of them is to yourself. Although the lump you have may be only a cyst, we cannot be sure of this without a biopsy. If it is a growth, you have a much better chance of avoiding a serious problem if you act now, no matter what the inconvenience. The added time may be the difference between a localized growth and one that has spread. Please consider carefully the idea of taking care of this first and your other business afterward." This type of statement, which leaves the patient in control and emphasizes the positive, is far better than one that uses scare tactics and paternalism such as, "That lump may be cancer. It must come out."

Yet a third situation presents another face of fear and anxiety.

A 60-year-old man is seen by a physician for abdominal pain. During the abdominal examination, the physician palpates a pulsatile mass that he thinks may be an abdominal aortic aneurysm. He explains to the patient that he would like to obtain an ultrasound examination of the abdomen to see if bulging of one of the great vessels is causing the pain. The patient says, "Come on, doctor. I don't want any tests. Just give me something for the pain." The physician tries to explain that this aneurysm might be hazardous for the patient and that it is very important to know if it is really there and, if so, how large it is. The patient becomes increasingly agitated. "Tests, tests, and more tests—that's all you guys know how to do. I just want some relief. You don't care about that—you want your tests."

In this situation, the physician must ask himself why the patient is so agitated. Why is he angry? Is there fear behind the anger—fear of not obtaining relief, fear of what may be found on the tests? Since the patient's primary concern is pain relief, the physician might say, "I will certainly give you something for the pain. However, in addition to treating the pain, it is important to treat whatever you have that may be causing the problem. We need to discover the source of the pain. Have you had a bad experience with certain tests?" The patient might answer, "A few years ago, I had a dye test for my kidneys, and it nearly killed me. They beat on my chest." This would give the physician a chance to respond, "Now I understand why you feel so strongly about testing. I don't blame you." The physician can then go on and carefully explain the benign nature and importance of ultrasound.

In this scenario, the patient's fears led him to be negative, almost hostile. The physician had to forge an alliance with the patient (in effect, remove himself as a source of the fear and join the patient in an effort to solve the problem). He accomplished this by meeting the patient's primary demand, pain control, and then acknowledging and exploring the patient's strongly negative response to the physician's suggestions.

Fear and Anxiety
About Specific Procedures
or Operations

There is some information available to help the physician understand a patient's reactions to a physical threat such as a surgical procedure. In general, patients show regressive patterns. They tend to
draw on defense mechanisms useful to them in childhood. These
may differ in different patients. Some may become very docile and
obedient. Behind this is the assumption that good behavior will net
them a reward, a good outcome. Others will act with bravado, denying fear. Often these patients are merely allying themselves with
the physician and thereby denying the potential danger they face. It
has been shown that a moderate amount of anxiety is useful,
whereas too much or too little is not. When fear is too great, it carries over into the recovery period, no matter what the result, ham-
pering return to normal life. When fear is too small, the patient may
develop anger for whatever pain or inconvenience has occurred,
and thus again not do well during follow-up. In order to achieve a
useful but not crippling amount of anxiety, it is important for the
physician to explain the dangers involved in a particular illness or
procedure and what will be done about them. It is also essential to
forewarn the patient about things such as pain or devices such as
the respirator. Thorough explanations help the patient do what has
been called "the useful work of worrying." As discomfort arises,
the patient is prepared for it, rather than panicking or thinking
something has gone wrong. An example follows:

A basically healthy 72-year-old man enters the hospital for repair of an in-
guinal hernia. His physician reassures him that it is a minor operation and
that he will be home in 3 or 4 days. The operation goes well. Several hours
after the operation, the patient is given a little clear liquid to drink. He
begins to swallow it but suddenly feels very nauseated and retches. He experiences a searing pain in the area of the surgery. The thought of some
serious complication goes through his head, and he begins to perspire and
feel light-headed. A nurse reassures him, gives him an antiemetic, and increases the rate of the intravenous fluid. Later, he tries to void but cannot.
Again he becomes frightened. He thinks, "That SOB surgeon said it was a
minor operation."

This case illustrates a problem of postoperative anxiety and
anger, which could easily have been avoided. The patient might
have been told about nausea after anesthesia and what could be
done about it. He could have been told about early pain. He could
have been warned that men in his age range sometimes have diffi-

culty voiding and need urinary catheterization. Rather than implying that the operation was simple, the physician could have informed the patient about different problems that are common, not serious, but nevertheless uncomfortable. The steps that could be taken to remedy them could also have been explained. This would have produced a calmer and more grateful postoperative patient.

In addition to planned procedures, there are numerous medical situations in which specific fears can be anticipated. A few examples are acute myocardial infarction in a young person with its attendant threat to earning power and normal family life, breast cancer in a young woman with its accompanying threat of disfigurement and disruption of normal sexual relationships, and amputation in any age group, bringing with it the specter of immobility and dependency. When patients present with illnesses such as these, it is useful to confront these fears immediately and not wait for them to smolder and grow. For example, in a first or second encounter with a patient in the coronary care unit, the physician might say, "You are probably wondering what this will do to your job, your ability to engage in normal activities." Many times, it is simply enough to let the patient know that the majority of patients return to normal function and that special programs are available to help with this. Patients will appreciate the fact that the physician is "tuned in" to their fears and will be reassured by previewed solutions to possible problems. This anticipatory care can avert much emotional suffering.

Physicians are made anxious by particular situations or patients also. Each physician must try to recognize her or his own vulnerable areas and deal with them honestly. This may involve additional training or turning to one's colleagues for help. The important point is self-awareness and action in the best interest of the patient.

Panic Disorder

Sometimes anxiety itself is the major medical problem. A formal classification of anxiety has been agreed upon and is reviewed in one of the suggested readings (Brown, 1984). We discuss here one specific diagnosis: panic disorder, an illness characterized by random attacks of fear and apprehension, with physical symptoms including dyspnea, palpitations, choking sensations, dizziness, paresthesias, hot and cold flashes, and psychologic symptoms including fear of dying or of going crazy. Three attacks in a 3-week period, not provoked by exertion or by a threatening situation, are necessary for the diagnosis. It is most common in women, often begins in the early twenties, lasts throughout life, and drives patients to multiple physicians, none of whom can pinpoint a physical problem. It is important to recognize the condition and to refer the patient to someone skilled in psychopharmacology, since tricyclics and monoamine oxidose (MAO) inhibitors are often useful in the management of this condition.

Pharmacotherapy

Most pharmacologic agents used in the treatment of anxiety are central nervous system (CNS) depressants. Alcohol is the most commonly used nonprescription agent employed in this way. The benzodiazepines were introduced in 1960 and have become the most widely prescribed agents in the treatment of anxiety (Table 13-1). Although many benzodiazepines are available, the clinical differences among them are rather modest. Certain general rules apply to their use, no matter which agent is chosen:

1. Patients who use benzodiazepines round the clock and for periods of more than a few months may develop both tolerance, necessitating escalated dosages, and physical dependence, calling for formal withdrawal protocols. Therefore, where possible, use should be restricted to "when necessary," or once to twice per day during a difficult emotional period.

2. Benzodiazepines, like alcohol, have a disinhibiting effect, and occasionally cause agitation or loss of behavioral control. This should be watched for in all patients, but particularly in elderly people or those with organic brain syndromes.

3. Alcohol enhances the CNS depressant effect of the benzodiazepines.

4. Benzodiazepines have a muscle relaxant action that may, in part, explain the relief of symptoms of anxiety. Small dosages may be used for this purpose (e.g., in patients with low back pain).

5. Benzodiazepines should be used in conjunction with, not instead of, supportive interpersonal care.

A 57-year-old woman reports intermittent chest pain unrelated to activity. A stress test is negative, and the patient is reassured. She continues to ex-

Table 13-1. Widely used agents for treatment of fear and anxiety

Drug	Average single dose*	Interval	Elimination
Chlordiazepoxide (Librium), 1960	10 mg	1–4 times/day	Slow
Diazepam (Valium), 1961	5 mg	1–4 times/day	Slow
Oxazepam (Serax), 1963	15 mg	1–4 times/day	Int to rapid
Clorazepate (Tranxene), 1974	7.5 mg	1–4 times/day	Slow
Lorazepam (Ativan), 1977	1–2 mg	1–4 times/day	Int
Alprazolam (Xanax), 1981	0.5 mg	1–4 times/day	Int

Int = intermediate.
*These dosages should be halved for some individuals, such as the elderly or other sensitive patients.

perience pain and is seen in the emergency room on numerous occasions without objective cardiac abnormalities. On one of these visits, she admits to multiple life stresses in the last few months. "I manage a home-decorating store and deal continually with difficult business problems. My husband is going through a difficult period; he has several phobias. Both my children are having marital problems. My elderly mother lives next door and depends on me for everything. I can't do it all!" The patient is visibly shaky. Her palms are moist. Her face is drawn. The physician speaks to her about obtaining some counseling to help her set limits and cope with her situational problems. He begins her on alprazolam, 0.5 mg twice per day, with the clear understanding that it is not a solution, but a *temporary aid* to be accompanied by formal psychologic help. She obtains counseling and, over a few months, has less pain and begins to regain control over her life. The alprazolam is reduced to a prn dosage.

Summary

Anxiety is ever present in physician-patient relations. It presents many faces and requires a variety of responses. Neither ignoring it nor handling it with blanket reassurance is adequate. At times, what is needed is to give the patient more information; at other times, the key is more patient control. Sometimes a specific fear is present and must be dealt with; at other times, hidden sources of fear need to be revealed. Occasionally, anxiety itself is the illness and will require treatment as such. Although medications are available and can be very useful in lessening anxiety, time and a caring attitude are almost always the mainstays of treatment. It helps to remember those things that produce fear and anxiety in all of us: the prospect of pain, disability, loss of identity and independence, and of course, death. When fears can be anticipated, it is better to deal with them openly rather than waiting until they are manifest. If prevention fails, treatment of emotional suffering is as worthy as treatment of physical suffering.

Suggested Reading

Brown, J. T., Mulrow, C. D., and Stoudemire, A. G. The anxiety disorders. *Ann. Intern. Med.* 100:558, 1984.

Greenblatt, D. J., Shader, R. I., and Abernathy, D. R. Current status of benzodiazepines. *N. Engl. J. Med.* 309:354, 1983.

Janis, I. L. *Psychologic Stress.* New York: Wiley, 1958.

Kandel, E. R. From metapsychology to molecular biology: Explorations into the nature of anxiety. *Am. J. Psychiatry* 140:1277, 1983.

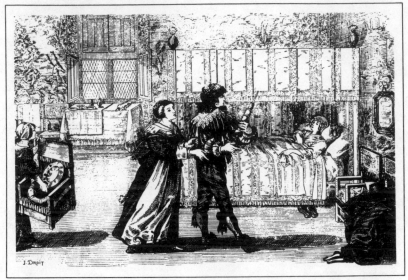

A physician prepares an enema syringe for a wealthy patient. A serving maid brings in a bedside commode. The clothing is typical of the period (reign of Louis XIII). (Engraving by Abraham Bosse, 1602–1676.)

14. Procedures

Medical students and house officers are often enthusiastic about performing diagnostic and therapeutic procedures. Successful performance of such techniques is regarded as proof that the individual is acquiring the requisite skills of an experienced physician. Of course, nothing could be further from the truth since many procedures can be skillfully performed by paramedical personnel who may lack complete understanding of many aspects of clinical practice.

Other features of procedures that often lead to their popularity are the ease and extent of reimbursement for such techniques by health care insurance plans. It is well known among clinicians that a diagnostic or therapeutic procedure requiring 30 to 40 minutes of physician time may entitle the physician to a fee in excess of $1,000, while 1 hour of painstaking questioning and examining a patient may be rewarded with $100 or less.

Such educational and economic facets of medical procedures can lead to severe ethical dilemmas in their performance: Under what circumstances can a medical student or young physician learn a procedure? Should all procedures be performed by experienced clinicians? How can a physician be objective in deciding when or if a patient needs a particular procedure given that the physician stands to gain so much by performing the procedure?

These ethical concerns as well as others have caused changes in the attitudes of physicians regarding the performance of procedures. The previously held medical student procedure doctrine, See one, do one, teach one, no longer holds. It is unfair and indefensible to expose a patient to the increased risk of complications in order to satisfy this doctrine. Current medical school policy in the United States requires careful instruction and constant supervision by experienced clinicians for students performing simple procedures. More complex techniques are reserved for residents or even subspecialty fellows, again under strict supervision. Many residency programs keep records concerning the number of procedures performed and the expertise demonstrated by members of the house staff. This allows the residency director to detect deficient performance of a specific procedure by a resident who can then receive remedial instruction.

When a procedure is performed by a less experienced physician under the close personal supervision of a more experienced colleague, the risk to the patient is minimized. Young physicians must be given an opportunity to learn such techniques if the performance of these procedures is to continue. It is difficult to say how many procedures of a particular type need to be performed by a physician before he or she is qualified as experienced at that procedure.

To some degree, each residency director and even each individual physician must decide when a particular procedure is performed with adequate skill. This is not a simple and straightforward decision since, as already noted, physicians may profit greatly by performing procedures. Therefore, it is not surprising that widely accepted indications have arisen for the performance of various procedures. When a particular clinical situation meets one or more of the criteria listed as indications, then the physician *may* consider performing the procedure if no contraindications exist. Let us consider an example:

A 45-year-old woman is admitted to a coronary care unit because of severe chest pain. The electrocardiogram reveals that the patient has sustained an acute inferior wall myocardial infarction. Thirty-six hours after admission to the coronary care unit, the patient develops hypotension and a decrease in urine output. The attending physicians consider inserting a pulmonary arterial catheter for diagnosis (is the hypotension due to hypovolemia or incipient cardiogenic shock?) and management (monitor the hemodynamic response to volume administration).

Table 14-1 lists the commonly accepted indications for insertion of pulmonary arterial catheters. This clinical situation satisfies a criterion, and the catheter is inserted. It is important to convince oneself that a procedure is definitely indicated before it is performed. If complications arise during or after the procedure, both the physician and the patient understand why the risks were incurred.

The decision to perform or not to perform an indicated procedure is based on an analysis of potential risks and benefits accompanying the technique. This decision-making process and the technical skills required for the procedure both depend on the physician's experience. Decision-making and technical skills cannot be learned from textbook or journal reading alone. Hands-on experience in the clinical setting is required. It often takes years of clinical experience before a physician is expert in decision making and the technical performance of procedures. Young physicians may feel

*Table 14-1. Commonly accepted indications
for insertion of a pulmonary arterial catheter*

1. Management of complicated myocardial infarction
   a. Hypovolemia versus cardiogenic shock
   b. Ventricular septal rupture versus acute mitral regurgitation
   c. Severe left ventricular failure
   d. Right ventricular infarction
   e. Unstable angina
   f. Refractory ventricular tachycardia
2. Determination of cause of dyspnea and hypoxia (severe pulmonary disease versus left ventricular failure)
3. Assessment of afterload reduction therapy in patients with left ventricular failure
4. Differential diagnosis of shock (e.g., pulmonary embolism, heart failure, sepsis, hemorrhage, dehydration)
5. Assessment of possible cardiac tamponade (measurement of right ventricular function and filling pressures)
6. Management of postoperative open-heart surgical patients
7. Management of critically ill medical patients with associated cardiovascular disease
   a. Gastrointestinal hemorrhage
   b. Sepsis
   c. Respiratory failure
   d. Renal failure
8. Management of critically ill surgical patients with associated cardiovascular disease during noncardiac surgery

From J. M. Gore, J. S. Alpert, J. R. Benotti, P. W. Kotilainen, and C. I. Haffajee. *Handbook of Hemodynamic Monitoring.* Boston: Little, Brown, 1985. With permission.

distraught because this process seems difficult. It *is* difficult, and it is one of the reasons that many years of postgraduate medical training is required. Clinical medicine is analagous to professional sports: Many years of experience, practice, and sharpening of one's skills are required to produce outstanding performance.

A final point needs to be stressed concerning the performance of procedures: Any act that requires coordination and dexterity is more likely to be performed correctly if the operator has confidence in his or her ability to carry out the procedure successfully. Approaching procedures with the attitude "here goes nothing" guarantees a poor outcome. This is another reason for medical students and young physicians to perform procedures under the guidance and with the assistance of a senior colleague. Patients can sense a physician's lack of confidence, and this may lead to unnecessary anxiety on the part of both patient and physician. Only after the physician feels confident that he or she can perform the procedure without difficulty should the technique be performed without supervision or assistance. It is only at that point that the physician can feel comfortable about teaching one.

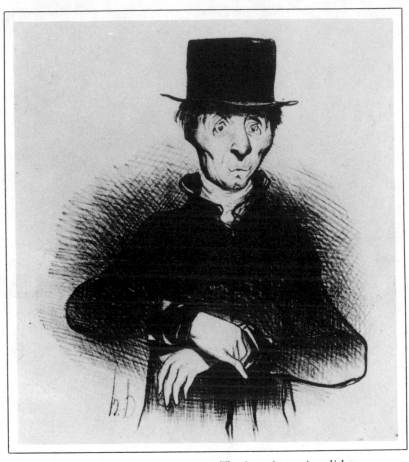

The imaginary invalid or hypochondriac says, "I'm done for . . . I'll have to make my will . . . they're going to bury me . . . farewell." (Lithograph by Honoré Daumier, 1808–1879.)

15. The So-called Difficult Patient

In general, physicians do not have the luxury of choosing only pleasant patients. The physician should be willing to try and help all comers. Only occasionally is the impasse so great that she or he must terminate the relationship. Usually the physician will attempt to overcome negative feelings in order to work with the patient. This may require considerable interpersonal skill.

A good deal has been written about patients with whom physicians are apt to have interpersonal difficulties. These writings have used various expressions: the difficult patient, the problem patient, the hateful patient. Although there clearly are patients who make things more difficult for the physician, there are also physician-related factors (e.g., biases, personal needs, and lack of interpersonal skills), which add to the difficulty of the situation. It is, therefore, useful to step back and look first at the physician's contribution to this problem.

Physician Biases

Surveys have suggested some *patient characteristics that many physicians find undesirable.* These attributes tend to cause a negative reaction in the physician, which may lessen her or his level of effort with that patient. Simply being aware of such biases may allow the physician to compensate and increase her or his efforts to try and help. Physicians often find patients with the following characteristics undesirable:

1. Patients who do not respect physician or respond to treatment
   a. Unappreciative
   b. Uncooperative
   c. Self-centered
   d. Manipulative
   e. Dependent
   f. Low pain threshold
   g. Unresponsive to treatment
   h. Terminal
2. Physically unattractive patients
   a. Disheveled or unkempt

   b. Markedly overweight
   c. Unpleasant odor
3. Self-destructive patients
   a. Suffering from drug overdose or habituated to drugs
   b. Suffering from alcohol intoxication or habituated to alcohol
   c. History of attempted suicide
4. Patients who communicate poorly
   a. Organic brain syndrome or memory-impaired
   b. Non-English-speaking
   c. Poor historian
   d. Reticent to relate symptoms

Cultural differences between physician and patient may also cause problems. The difficulty may arise because of differences in personal value systems or because physician and patient have different models of the disease process. A simple example follows:

A stoic 70-year-old presents to a physician with a broken rib. The physician tapes the area and gives the patient a prescription for pain. The patient says, "No, thanks. I don't need the pain medicine." The physician insists, "Take the prescription with you, just in case." The patient, who prides himself on never having taken so much as an aspirin for a headache, does not fill the prescription. He reacts to the physician's insistence as even more of a challenge to his willpower. The broken rib is very painful, and the patient splints that side, suppresses deep breathing, suppresses coughing, and develops pneumonia.

   The problem here is that the physician assumed the patient would respond to pain as the physician would—by taking medication. Thus, the physician did not explain the medical importance of minimizing the pain (i.e., to enable deep breathing and coughing). The patient saw the pain medication as a crutch. He viewed taking it as a defeat rather than as important treatment.
   The differences in personality and in illness model between physician and patient led to noncompliance and further medical problems. Such problems are common when the physician and patient stem from different cultures or live in very different social milieux. Therefore, it is important to be sure that the patient's understanding of the problem and the treatment match the physician's, and that differences in style and conceptual framework are worked out. A careful explanation by the physician as well as an invitation to the patient to ask questions will help. Specific questions as to the pa-

tient's understanding of the illness and the treatment represent an even better approach to this problem.

Physicians should be aware of their own personal biases. They have likes and dislikes that may interfere with patient care. One physician may be annoyed by meek, cowering patients. Another may be more aggravated by patients with bravado. The important point is to be aware and to try and realize that the patient need not be taken into one's circle of close friends: She or he is simply seeking help. As with the list of generally held biases, the physician may not be able to change her or his preferences, but may be able to minimize their effects.

A gender difference may also cause problems between physician and patient. Some patients may feel more comfortable with a physician of the same gender; others may prefer the opposite; still others may have trouble responding to a physician because of gender. This may be due to what or whom the patient is accustomed, his or her upbringing or cultural background—any of a number of factors. Physicians may have similar preferences or prejudices. They must be aware of and sensitive to their own as well as their patients' preferences and prejudices, since these can drastically affect physician-patient relationships and certain aspects of treatment and diagnosis.

Emotion-Handling Skills

Patients who are difficult to deal with may be so because of strong emotions such as anger, frustration, or sadness. It is important for the physician to recognize these emotions and to help the patient deal with them. Dr. Julien Bird and Dr. Steven Cohen-Cole, in some unpublished work, make some useful suggestions in this regard.

To begin with, the physician's nonverbal behavior is important. If one wants to communicate warmth when trying to share some distress, it may help to move closer to patients, at times to touch them. On the other hand, if one is trying to cool down anger, it is better to move away, to lower one's voice, and to avoid provoking the patient in any way.

Several verbal behaviors are useful in handling emotions. Statements seem to be more effective than questions when dealing with feelings. Saying "You seem angry" is usually much more productive than "Why are you angry?" Bird and Cohen-Cole have broken down emotion-handling skills into several steps:

1. *Empathy.* Put yourself in the patient's position; try to feel the emotion; name the emotion. "You seem angry."

2. *Understanding.* Express your understanding for the patient's emotion. "I can understand why this situation would make you angry." Sometimes partial self-disclosure (i.e., "When I had a similar problem, I was angry.") will be helpful.

3. *Respect.* Find some area in which you can express respect for the patient. For example, say, "You really have handled this difficult problem admirably."

4. *Support.* State your intention to be of help. "I am here to help you. Together we should be able to improve your situation."

There are certain disruptive verbal behaviors that we are all tempted to use. Examples of these include

1. Aggravating questions: "Why are you so impatient?"
2. Inappropriate reassurance: "Everything will be fine."
3. Paternalistic scolding: "It is foolish for you to be so negative."

The following cases attempt to illustrate a few of the more helpful and less helpful behaviors.

A 59-year-old woman sees a physician for exertional chest pain. A stress test is markedly positive, and the physician suggests coronary angiography. The patient turns pale. Tears begin to form in her eyes. She stares at the physician, her hands grasping the sides of her chair. The physician says, "Don't worry, you'll be fine. The test is no big deal." She begins to sob.

In this report, the physician glossed over the patient's feelings with a vague statement of reassurance. He or she might have said, "I can understand how the idea of cardiac catheterization is frightening. Most people are very anxious about it [an empathetic statement]." "However, if you'll let me, I'll explain it more thoroughly, and you'll see that it is not painful or dangerous. I think I can put to rest some of your fears. From what I know of you, I think you'll handle it very well [an affirmation of respect], and I'll certainly do my best to help you with it [a pledge of support]."

A businessman is being treated by a physician for hypertension. This interchange occurs during the visit. The physician asks, "How are you doing, Mr. K?" The patient responds, "Lousy." The physician says, "I'm sorry to hear that." The patient blurts out, "This is the fourth medicine I've had in 2 months! The first made me dizzy. The second nauseated me. The third dried my mouth out. This one has ruined my sex life. What am I, some kind of guinea pig for your various poisons?" The physician answers, "You've really had a terrible time [an empathetic statement]! It's no wonder you're angry [naming the emotion]. It's been very good of you to try several drugs, considering the difficulties they have caused you [an expression of respect]. It is obviously not easy to find the best medication. However, it is very important to control your blood pressure. I'm convinced that if we work together we can do it. Certainly I'd like to continue trying [a statement of support]."

In this report, the patient was angry about medication side effects. Undoubtedly the physician was frustrated too. It would have been a great temptation for the physician to say something like "Some people are difficult to treat," thereby shifting the blame onto the patient. This would probably have heightened the patient's anger and anxiety. Instead, the physician chose to help the patient handle his anger and to continue offering support. This is much more apt to see the two through a difficult period.

Difficult Patient Types
Certain personality types appear to be particularly difficult for physicians. A few of these are described since it may be useful to recognize them and to have some plan for helping them.

ENTITLED DEMANDERS
These patients will make unreasonable demands sound legitimate and will play on the physician's conscientiousness to try and obtain what the patient wants. In this situation, the physician must recognize and explain to the patient that he or she is entitled to good medical care, but not necessarily to his or her particular requests. An example follows:

A 64-year-old man who had a triple coronary bypass graft operation 8 years ago is admitted with recurrent angina pectoris. The patient is stabilized, and coronary angiography is scheduled. Unfortunately, the cardiologist with whom the patient identifies most closely is about to leave on a vacation. Since the patient is stable, the angiography could easily be postponed for the 10 days in which the physician is away. The cardiologist explains this to the patient. She also points out that one of her associates could do the angiogram in her absence. The patient becomes indignant. "How can you do this to me, doctor? I heard that you were the best. I want the best, not some substitute." The cardiologist again explains to the patient that it appears safe to wait if he will just follow some reasonable constraints. "That's impossible! I have a business to run. I need to know where I stand now. Where is the dedication doctors used to have? I never let my vacations interfere with my obligations. My chest is beginning to hurt now because you have upset me so much."

This is obviously a complex problem. The physician is about to leave on one of her all too rare vacations. The patient is making her feel irresponsible. Yet if she does not leave on time, she will compromise time that she very much needs for herself. The physician must first help the patient handle his anger and then point out what the patient is and what he is not entitled to. He deserves good care but not his particular demands.

"Mr. L., I can understand why you are upset. It is very disappointing for you to have to wait or to have someone who knows you less well do the angiogram. It is important to me that you get excellent care, and I will see to it that you get it. However, it is impossible for me to follow your schedule. If it is important to you to have me do the angiogram, you must wait 10 days. Every indication is that this would be safe given your current medications and some activity limitation. If your business demands are such that the test must be now, I will arrange for an excellent person to do the angiogram."

This is all that the physician can do. If she accedes to the patient's demands, she jeopardizes her own family life. Only in an emergency, where no one else capable is present, should the physician give in to such a demand.

DEPENDENT CLINGERS

These patients overutilize the physician's services to the point where the physician dreads hearing from or seeing them. Often they begin by flattering the physician, showing unwarranted gratitude (i.e., they attempt to seduce the physician into giving them special care). However, as the calls and visits begin to pile up, the physician's initial positive reaction turns to annoyance and her or his behavior to avoidance.

There are some steps one can take to lessen the problem. First, since the cause of the patient's behavior is a sense of helplessness and profound dependence, avoidance on the part of the physician only intensifies the patient's efforts to win the physician's attention. It may be helpful to recognize the patient's special needs by giving them some special care. One way to do this is to assure the patient that one understands the patient's need for close observation and to set up a schedule of relatively frequent, even if brief, appointments so that the patient will not have to use a variety of other mechanisms to see the physician. At the same time, one can gently but firmly set down some rules about calls or drop-in visits by explaining one's inability to respond to certain demands.

MANIPULATIVE HELP-REJECTERS
These patients return again and again to report that their treatment did not work. When one symptom disappears, another appears. Their pessimism increases proportionally to the physician's enthusiasm about any particular regimen. The physician begins to dread the visits in a manner similar to the way she or he dreads the dependent clinger.

Once again, the patient's behavior usually stems from a fear of abandonment. Thus, the more the physician withdraws, the more symptomatic the patient will become. In this setting, the best plan may be to acknowledge the failure of the treatment, share the pessimism, and emphasize the physician-patient relationship, rather than the success of a given program with its implied termination of the relationship. An example follows:

A 64-year-old woman is under treatment for a functional gastrointestinal complaint. Careful work-up reveals no abnormality, and not surprisingly, several medications have been ineffective in relieving her symptoms. The physician initially tries reassurance. "At least we know nothing serious is wrong with your stomach." The patient answers, "You know, in the last few weeks, I have had terrible headaches too." After several symptom changes (the latest being back pain) and negative work-ups, the physician tries a new approach. "It must be very difficult for you to do the work you do with those back pains. I will give you some medication. However, even more importantly, I would like to see you more frequently so that I can be of as much help as possible with this problem."

The key to handling this patient was to assure her that she would get care regardless of symptom outcome, thus defusing her anxiety about losing the physician. Any real enthusiasm about a possible cure causes this type of patient to fear termination of the physician-patient relationship.

Terminating the Relationship with a Patient
Rarely, a physician feels that she or he can no longer work productively with a patient. Aside from emergency circumstances, the

physician has the right to inform the patient that she or he can no longer assume responsibility for the patient's care. When possible, this should be done kindly. "I don't feel I'm being as helpful to you as I'd like to be. I would like you to find another physician. I will of course provide that person with your records." If the physician feels strongly, she or he should not back down even if the patient objects. It is difficult to provide good care when the physician has such strong negative feelings. The relationship is not officially terminated until the physician sends a registered letter stating that he or she "will provide emergency care until (usually 2 weeks), and after that will no longer be responsible for the patient's care." The registered letter documents the termination. The grace period allows the patient time to find another physician.

Summary

It is curious that our medical training lauds us for solving difficult medical problems but devotes so little time to difficult interpersonal situations. Surely difficult interpersonal problems are as common as complex medical dilemmas. In this chapter, we reviewed some aspects of difficult physician-patient interactions. We would like to emphasize that these are two-way problems. Biases, personal needs, cultural differences, and the interpersonal skill of the physician contribute to such problems. There are patients who are particularly troublesome to deal with, but some skills are available to cope with these individuals. It is possible and very satisfying to improve one's ability to deal with the so-called difficult patient.

Suggested Reading

Groves, J. E. Taking care of the hateful patient. *N. Engl. J. Med.* 298:883, 1978.

Kleinman, A., Eisenberg, L., and Good, B. Clinical lessons from anthropologic and cross cultural research. *Ann. Intern. Med.* 88:251, 1978.

Lipp, M. R., (ed.). Problem Patients. In *Respectful Treatment: The Human Side of Medical Care.* Hagerstown, Md.: Harper & Row, 1977. Pp. 108–123.

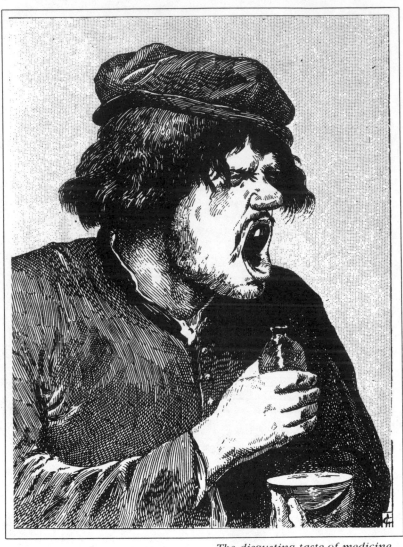

The disgusting taste of medicine. (Etching by Adrian Brouwer, 1606–1638.)

16. Malpractice

No subject creates greater fear and hostility among physicians than medical malpractice. A rather uncommon occurrence 30 or 40 years ago, malpractice suits are now everyday events. More than $1.5 billion are spent by American physicians on malpractice insurance premiums. Unfortunately, no physician, regardless of skill or training, is immune to malpractice litigation. Even though the physician may be convinced that he or she acted in the patient's best interest, it may not be so apparent to the patient or the patient's family. Many law firms specialize in medical malpractice cases, advertising on television or in the newspapers, eagerly seeking clients who feel they have been wronged. In such an environment, even the most skilled and compassionate physician may become the target of a malpractice suit.

There are many reasons for the remarkable increase in malpractice cases in recent years. The two most common explanations are (1) the disappearance of the close physician-patient relationship of previous years, and (2) the high cost of medical care and the resultant high expectations of patients and family. The unfortunate triad that often leads to malpractice litigation comprises a bad result, a big bill, and a poor physician-patient relationship. The patient and family expect a good result and are dismayed at the poor outcome; they are shocked by the large bill (even if it is being paid by an insurance company or Medicare); they are irritated by the physician. The end result of this constellation of circumstances is a malpractice suit.

There are five ways in which physicians commonly become defendants in malpractice litigation (Danner, 1984):

1. Through the physician's own negligence or failure to conform to generally accepted medical practice
2. Through the negligence or failings of secretaries, nurses, or physician's assistants working for the physician
3. Through the physician's failure to obtain adequate informed consent from the patient prior to diagnosis and treatment
4. Through a breach of the physician-patient social contract (i.e., abandoning the patient, inappropriately disclosing confidential information to others, guaranteeing a cure or a perfect result)
5. Through negligence of the physician's partners

Once a physician accepts a patient for treatment, the physician is obliged to provide care for the individual that conforms to norms of good medical practice. Physicians are held to the standard of their level of training. Thus, a general practitioner is compared to standards for other general practitioners, not standards for specialists. It is expected that physicians will keep up with advances in therapy and diagnosis so that they can adhere to advancing standards of care.

An error in judgment does not constitute grounds for a malpractice case as long as the error was not contrary to accepted standards of care. In addition, physicians must always act in good faith toward the patient (i.e., the physician must act with the patient's best interests at heart).

Patients deserve a thorough and understandable explanation of their illness and the diagnostic and therapeutic interventions that are being considered. Patients have the right to participate in the decision-making process concerning diagnosis and therapy. In most cases, however, patients accept the physician's judgment on which modalities should be employed.

Obtaining informed consent from the patient is a two-part process. First, the patient is *informed* concerning the risks and potential benefits of the planned diagnostic or therapeutic intervention. Alternative strategies are also discussed, and the physician explains why he or she feels that the suggested plan is better than alternative solutions. Second, the patient *consents* to the planned intervention orally or in writing.

Some physicians feel that in order to obtain informed consent, they must tell the patient of every conceivable risk and complication associated with the planned procedure. The result of such truth-telling is a terrified, distraught patient. Common sense dictates that this is poor medical practice. A preferable system for obtaining informed consent is as follows:

1. Sit at the patient's bedside and explain the nature of the patient's illness and the rationale for the planned procedure.
2. Note that all procedures are associated with some risk, although it is often quite small. Similarly, driving one's car on the highway is associated with a small but definite risk of death or disfigurement.
3. List the most common complications associated with the planned procedure. For example, cardiac catheterization is associated

with small but definite risks of myocardial infarction, stroke, arrhythmia, and even death.

4. Point out the potential benefit of the procedure to the patient as well as why this particular procedure is advised rather than alternative techniques.
5. Elicit any questions or doubts that the patient may have and respond to them.
6. Reassure the patient. Every one of us has anxieties when faced with potential risks to our health and our lives.
7. Leave a written informed consent form for the patient to read and sign at his or her leisure unless an emergency sitution is present.

Malpractice Prevention

The best way to deal with medical malpractice is to prevent it. A strong physician-patient relationship, tact, kindness, thoroughness, equity in billing, and concern for the welfare of the patient are factors that can prevent malpractice litigation. Physicians do not have to accept any and all patients who seek their attention. The physician may decide before undertaking a course of diagnosis and therapy that a particular patient's personality or attitude is such that a satisfactory relationship cannot be created. In this situation, the physician should calmly and tactfully decline involvement in the patient's care.

Finally, if the physician does become involved in a malpractice case, he or she should attempt to maintain equanimity. Often, the physician is involved as one small part of a larger group of individuals who are being sued (i.e., the hospital, all doctors who took any part in the patient's care, equipment manufacturers).

Do not take the litigation personally. Malpractice suits are rarely personal vendettas against the physician. Rather, they are attempts by an individual or a family to gain redress for actual or perceived injury from sources that seem to have limitless capital (i.e., the physician, the hospital, and the insurance company).

There is a list of dos and don'ts for physicians who have become involved in a malpractice suit (Danner, 1984). The dos include notifying the malpractice insurance company and cooperating fully with it and its lawyers, compiling all records and recollections about the incident, and before complying, discussing all requests for information or meetings from the patient or the patient's lawyer with one's own insurance company. Common prohibitions include altering the patient's records in any way, discussing the case with anyone except the assigned representatives of the insurance company, and overreaction against the patient and lawyers or court-appointed officials involved in the case.

Hopefully, advice on medical malpractice will never be needed. However, malpractice suits are very common, and the most compassionate and skilled physician may become embroiled in such an action, even when he or she is completely blameless. Try to practice the best, most humane medicine possible, and if a malpractice litigation does arise, let the insurance company and its lawyers handle it.

Suggested Reading
Danner, D. *Medical Malpractice: A Primer for Physicians.* Rochester, N.Y.: Lawyers Co-operative, 1984.

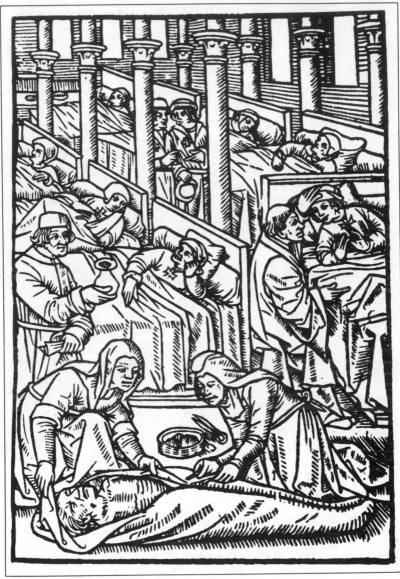

A medieval hospital with nuns sewing a corpse into a shroud and a physician examining urine in a flask. (From Jehan Petit's Saint Gelais, 1ᵉ Vergier d'Honneur.)

17. Disposition Problems

Every medical student, house officer, and physician knows the frustration of a patient who becomes a disposition problem. These patients are individuals who remain in the hospital beyond the time necessary for acute care because they have nowhere to go once they arc discharged.

Disposition problems often arise in elderly individuals who are too infirm to return home and who thus require nursing home placement. Many such patients have limited economic means or insurance coverage. Consequently, nursing homes are reluctant to accept such patients, fearing that reimbursement for services rendered will not be forthcoming. In some such cases, the patient has adequate insurance and private means to pay for nursing home residence but is so sick that he or she requires more intensive care than the nursing home can provide.

Another type of disposition problem involves a younger patient who has such severe disability that family members feel incapable of caring for the patient after discharge from the hospital. For example, a middle-aged patient with extensive central nervous system dysfunction might require constant attention not available at home. If such an individual lacks adequate financial resources to cover the cost of nursing home or chronic hospital residence, a disposition problem develops for the attending physician.

Other examples of disposition problems are indigent and even homeless individuals who come to the emergency room seeking care for a minor problem. Under normal circumstances, patients with minor problems are discharged to home from the emergency room following treatment. However, the physician and the hospital staff may be reluctant to discharge a patient from the emergency room if he or she has nowhere to go: A disposition problem has developed for the emergency room staff.

All of these patients have a common problem: They have no place to go following hospital discharge. Social workers are usually consulted at this point, and a search begins for a posthospital residence. Unfortunately, many patients are difficult to place either because of the high level of nursing care that is required or because the patient cannot afford to pay for such care. The patient no longer has an acute medical problem requiring hospitalization, but discharge is not possible. The patient remains in the hospital as a boarder. Such patients are often unwanted by the hospital since their insurance coverage may not be adequate for a prolonged hospitalization. Frustration often runs high for physicians, nurses, and administrative personnel involved with such patients. Tensions can lead to the use of pejorative terms with regard to these patients. Words like "gomer" (get out of my emergency room), "dump", or "turf" (transfer the patient to another service or facility) may be employed by the involved staff. These terms rob the patient of his or her humanity and may lead to unkind or unfeeling treatment by the physician and hospital staff. If the physician will stop for a moment and imagine what it feels like to have no place to go and to be unwanted even by medical personnel, it will be obvious that such attitudes and terms need to be avoided regardless of how frustrating the situation may be.

Solving disposition problems often requires imagination on the part of the physician (see App. B). Sometimes, a patient can be accepted at a facility with a lower level of nursing care than initially anticipated after further rehabilitation (physical and occupational therapy) at the acute care hospital. Alternatively, some patients can be discharged to home with extensive support from visiting nurses and home health aides. Social workers are knowledgeable about alternative disposition solutions. A few minutes' conversation between the attending physician and the social worker often produces a solution to a disposition problem:

An elderly man suffers a myocardial infarction complicated by arrhythmias and heart failure. Before entering the hospital, the patient lived with his infirm, semiinvalid wife in their own home. Previous to his myocardial infarction, the patient cared for his wife, performing most of the household chores and the cooking. During the patient's hospitalization, it becomes obvious to the attending physician, the nursing staff, and the members of the cardiac rehabilitation team that this independent man will have difficulty performing household chores and cooking because of his chronic left ventricular failure. It is suggested that both the patient and his wife be admitted to a nursing home, a solution that the patient vigorously opposes because of limited financial resources and loss of personal independence. The attending physician and the hospital staff confer with one of the institution's social workers. The social worker suggests arranging a program that entails a maximum of supportive services for the patient and his wife in their own home. Such services include frequent check-ups by the visiting nurse; three visits a week by a home health aide to assist the couple with housework, shopping, and cooking; delivery of meals by a senior citizen shut-in program; and transportation assistance for the patient and his wife from friends, family, and a senior citizen shuttle service. The patient accepts this solution, and a satisfactory home program is achieved.

In this scenario, the social worker's knowledge of available community resources prevented this patient from becoming a chronic disposition problem. This example underlines the fact that physicians need to be aware of resources in the hospital and in the community that can be employed to benefit their patients (see App. B).

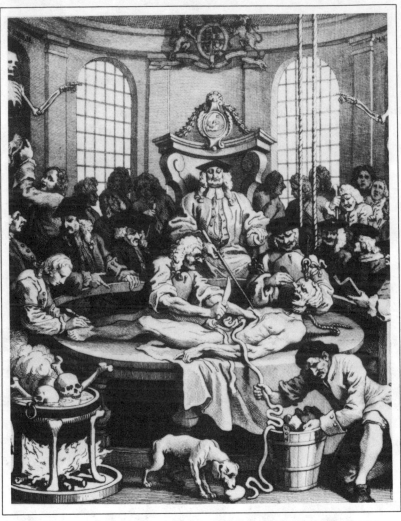

"The Reward of Cruelty." This
satiric engraving of a dissection
class in eighteenth-century England demonstrates that medical
education had changed little since
the fifteenth century (see Chap. 4).
The professor lectures pedantical-
ly, far removed from the actual
dissection, which is performed by
a prosector. (Engraving from 1751
by William Hogarth, 1697–1764.)

18. Autopsies

One of the most unpleasant tasks a physician must face is requesting permission from family members to perform an autopsy on a recently deceased relative. The task is unpleasant because it comes at a time when family and physician alike are grieving for the deceased. At this emotional moment, the physician must sometimes seek permission to examine the organs of the patient or even ask permission to obtain certain organs for transplantation.

Some religious sects believe that autopsy involves desecration of the body. Many other individuals feel that autopsy involves ghoulish mutilation of the body. At times, family members have not yet come to terms with the patient's death. They will say, "He has suffered enough." Clearly, the physician who is seeking autopsy permission must be sensitive to the attitudes and beliefs that exist in the deceased patient's family. Should the physician even bother to ask for autopsy permission? Is the information obtained useful? Both of these questions must be answered in the affirmative before the physician seeks the family's permission to perform an autopsy.

Traditional medical education of the eighteenth and nineteenth centuries often included a year spent performing autopsies. It was believed that the clinical-pathologic correlation learned by such an exercise increased the young physician's diagnostic acumen. Similar educational attitudes persisted into the twentieth century, and many older clinicians can point to a year of pathologic training as an important facet of their medical education. In the waning years of the twentieth century, however, universal training in pathology seems redundant to many medical educators. It is rather uncommon nowadays for a patient to die without the diagnosis of the fatal illness having been clearly established ante mortem. The extraordinary ability of computed tomography (CT) scans, angiograms, biopsies, nuclear scans, and ultrasound techniques to visualize pathologic alterations in form and function has led to the belief that the surprise revelation of the diagnosis during postmortem examination is largely a thing of the past. Yet one in 10 autopsies at a Harvard-affiliated hospital in 1960, 1970, and 1980 revealed a diagnosis that, if recognized while the patient lived, might have been lifesaving (Goldman, 1983).

The autopsy is not a useless academic exercise. First, pathologic confirmation of the diagnosis justifies the clinician's confidence in the diagnostic armamentarium and may reveal areas where either the clinicians or the diagnostic laboratories need strengthening. For example, incorrect identification of a tumor on a CT scan may point out the need to refine the technique or the interpretation of CT scans in the clinician's institution. Second, the clinician's understanding of a particular pathologic entity is often enhanced by a visual inspection of the diseased organs.

All postgraduate medical education programs have a conference for trainees that involves the presentation of pathologic material. A variety of formats are employed in such conferences. The traditional clinical pathologic conference (CPC) involves the presentation and discussion of a patient by a clinician who attempts to deduce the correct diagnosis. The climax of the CPC involves the revelation of the correct diagnosis by the pathologist. This exercise is often rather artificial, with both clinician and pathologist resorting to gamesmanship and pedantry in the course of the conference. A more useful pathologic teaching exercise is the morbidity and mortality conference, during which a number of clinicians comment on various features of the patient's clinical course, and the pathologist comments on the pathology and pathophysiology involved in the particular patient's disease. Less confrontational and pedantic, the morbidity and mortality conference is rapidly replacing the older CPC in most teaching hospitals. Thus, pathologic teaching is still an important part of postgraduate medical education, having been integrated into most medical and surgical training programs. Postmortem examinations supply material for these important teaching exercises.

At times, the autopsy examination can reveal errors in diagnostic or therapeutic reasoning or procedure. For example, the postmortem examination may disclose a previously unsuspected complication of a surgical or diagnostic procedure that played an important role in the patient's demise. The postmortem examination may also suggest new diseases or new connections among known diseases. Finally, by providing some estimate of the correspondence between the death certificate and the pathologic anatomy, the postmortem can help physicians interpret disease-specific mortality rates derived from death certificates.

Whenever possible, the autopsy should be requested by the physician who has been the most closely involved in the care of the patient. Consent for autopsy examination is obtained from the patient's legal next of kin. The hierarchy of priority in terms of granting permission is as follows:

1. Spouse
2. Adult son or daughter
3. Either parent
4. Adult brother or sister
5. The guardian of the deceased patient at the time of death
6. Any other person authorized or under legal obligation to dispose of the remains

Thus, if the deceased patient's spouse is either dead or incapable of granting permission for an autopsy (e.g., senile or in a coma), this responsibility falls on the shoulders of an adult son or daughter. It is not necessary for the physician to obtain permission from all members of a family group. For example, the physician may deal with one adult son or daughter of the patient. This individual would then be requested to notify other family members about the postmortem examination. The physician should be reasonably confident that other family members have been informed and have no objections at the time of the autopsy.

It is important for the physician to be certain that the person giving consent to the autopsy is actually the legal next of kin. For example, despite couple separations without divorce, the spouse is still legally next of kin. The physician should explain the purpose of the autopsy to the next of kin in as kindly a fashion as possible. The advantage to the family should be stressed (i.e., an autopsy will confirm and clarify the cause of death for family health records). Such information may be of importance in the medical care of surviving family members.

If at all possible, the autopsy request should be made in person, in a quiet place. It sometimes helps to be accompanied by a nurse who knows the family. However, the number of medical people should not be larger than this. The fact of death should often be announced gently and simply to avoid delaying and heightening anxiety. For example, a sensitive physician's request for postmortem examination might be, "I am very sorry but your father has died." If the final event occurred without much pain (fortunately, often the case in hospitals), one might say, "He did not suffer at the end." If the illness was a long and difficult one, it might be helpful to say, "She has been ill for such a long time. Perhaps it is a blessing in some ways that her ordeal is over." At this point, it helps to sit with the person, put one's hand on his or her hand or shoulder if appropriate, and allow him or her to express any emotions. Once the relative has had a chance to react and has settled down, one might say, "All of us wish as you do that we could have cured this illness. I know this is a very difficult time for you, but I would like to ask your permission to perform an autopsy. The information obtained from such an examination might be valuable for your family and would certainly benefit future patients with this illness. If you give permission for the autopsy, I will write to you and report the details of the examination for your family health records."

Family members are often concerned that the autopsy will delay or interfere with funeral arrangements. This is not the case at all. Indeed, pathology departments are very sensitive to this issue and work closely with funeral directors to prevent any delay or difficulty with the funeral. This should be pointed out to the family. At times, family members have strong negative feelings about examining certain areas of the deceased patient's body—for example, the brain. In such circumstances, the autopsy may exclude or even be limited to examination of specific organ systems (e.g., the heart and lungs in a patient dying of cardiovascular disease or the kidneys in a patient dying of renal disease).

If no family members are present at the time of the patient's demise, and it is not easy to call them into the hospital, the physician may choose to request autopsy permission over the telephone. When telephone permission is obtained, another person (not the telephone operator) must listen on an extension phone to witness the granting of autopsy permission.

A special document, known as a postmortem examination permission form, is filled out by the physician and signed by the family member granting autopsy permission as well as by the physician. When autopsy permission is obtained over the telephone, both the physician and the witness who listened to the consent for autopsy should sign a postmortem permission form. Figure 18-1 is a typical postmortem permission form. Restrictions should be specifically stated, or their absence should be acknowledged. In addition to this form, most pathology departments request a synopsis of the patient's clinical course to assist the pathologist in determining organ systems for special attention. Some hospitals have a separate form for the attending physician or house officer to fill out. Typically, such forms request the following information: clinical diagnosis, features requiring particular investigation or dissection, other relevant features of the clinical course, recent surgery or invasive procedures, history of tuberculosis or other infectious diseases, use of radioactive substances, and life-support systems (i.e., ventilator, dialysis) connected to the patient at the time of the patient's demise.

Permission for Postmortem Examination

Date: _____   Patient's Name: _____

Time of Death: _____   Address: _____

Attending Physician: _____   Birthdate/Age: _____

_____   Hospital Number: _____

1. I am the _____ of the deceased and entitled to control the disposition of the remains.
2. I, being the next of kin, of age and competent, request and authorize the medical staff of the Medical Center to perform a postmortem examination on the body of_____
3. I, being the next of kin, am unaware that any other person, in the same class of relationship as I, has expressed any contrary intentions.
4. I, being the next of kin, authorize the removal and retention or use of such organs and tissues as the physicians deem proper for diagnostic, scientific, and therapeutic purposes.
5. I, being the next of kin, authorize a full and complete postmortem examination with the following modifications/restrictions:

No restrictions: _____

Restrictions (please specify):

_____

Other considerations (please specify):

_____

_____

Signed: _____   Signed: _____
                                                (Witness)
Comments and/or extenuating circumstances regarding authorization for consent:

_____

_____

Telephone or verbal permission given from: _____

Witness 1: _____

Witness 2: _____

Fig. 18-1. Postmortem permission form employed at the University of Massachusetts Medical Center, Worcester, Massachusetts.

When possible, cannulas and other disposable devices should be left attached to the patient until the autopsy.

The physician must be aware that the death of certain patients involves medicolegal issues that make the autopsy mandatory. Such postmortem examinations are performed by the medical examiner.

Table 18-1. Common situations that may
require a postmortem examination by the medical examiner

1. Violent or accidental deaths
2. Death outside of hospital (e.g., at home or at work)
3. Sudden or unexpected deaths within or outside of hospital, including death during childbirth or abortion, death in the operating
   room, or death in a mental clinic or hospital
4. Drug- or alcohol-related deaths, including deaths of drug addicts
5. Death of an individual in jail or in police custody
6. Death within 24 hours of admission to the hospital
7. Death involving features suspicious of homicide (e.g., suspected poi-
   soning)
8. Suspected suicide or death as a result of drug overdose
9. Death involving severe misconduct or malfeasance on the part of the
   hospital or clinicians
10. Individual states that require a postmortem examination by the
    medical examiner for specific conditions (e.g., many states require
    such an examination in patients who die of the sudden infant death
    syndrome)

Examples include patients who have died as the result of a gun-shot
wound or a motor vehicle accident. Such individuals almost invariably require a postmortem examination by the medical examiner with a subsequent coroner's inquest into the cause of the
patient's demise (Table 18-1). In such cases, the physician does *not*
seek autopsy permission from the family. Rather, he or she informs
the medical examiner's office about the details of the patient's
death. If the medical examiner's office decides that medicolegal issues are *not* a factor in this particular individual's death, then the attending physician can request autopsy permission from the family.
If the medical examiner desires an autopsy, then arrangements are
made by that individual to perform the autopsy; permission of next
of kin is not required.

It is, of course, most important that the physician subsequently
write or call the family member who granted permission for the
autopsy. Such letters could contain a brief description in layperson's terms of the results of the autopsy as well as the medical
name for the cause of death. For example, one might inform family
members that their relative "had died of a massive heart attack,
which in medical terms is called an extensive myocardial infarction." Such letters are invariably saved by relatives of the deceased

and serve as useful documentation for subsequent family health histories.

Suggested Reading

Goldman, L., Sayson, R., Robbins, S., Cohn, L. H., Bettmann, M., and Weisberg, M. The value of the autopsy in three medical eras. *N. Engl. J. Med.* 308:1000, 1983.

Schmidt, S. Consent for autopsies. *J.A.M.A.* 250:1161, 1983.

Schneiderman, H., and Gruhn, J. How and why to request an autopsy. *Postgrad. Med.* 77:153, 1985.

IV. Medical
Ethics

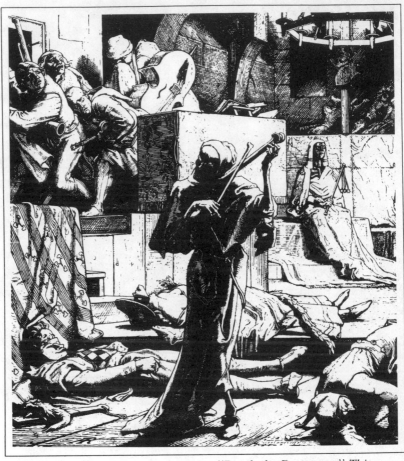

"Death the Destroyer." This frightening appearance of death at a masked ball reminds one of Poe's story, "The Mask of the Red Death." (Wood engraving by Steinbrecher after Alfred Rethel, 1816–1859.)

19. Medical Ethics, Medicine, and Literature

Medical Ethics

Many of the important social and ethical questions of our century relate to technologic developments in biomedical science: Is it appropriate to alter an individual's genetic makeup? When and for what indications should abortion be performed? Should euthanasia be available to terminally ill patients? What constitutes legal death? How vigorous should therapy be pursued in terminally ill patients? These questions have no right or wrong answers. Thoughtful men and women disagree on the answers to these complex problems. It is not uncommon to find disagreement among attending physicians, house officers, and nurses concerning the appropriate course of therapy in a critically or terminally ill patient. Many of these issues concern individuals outside the medical profession. Not only have medical professionals and patients debated these issues and continue to do so, but social agencies have as well. Elected and appointed legal and political officials play an important role in making these ethical decisions. For example, in 1973, within our memory, the judicial approach to therapeutic abortion has been altered, thereby changing the practicing physician's options.

Physicians have a responsibility to educate the public concerning the biomedical aspects of a particular ethical issue. Clearly, physicians often feel strongly about such issues, favoring one or another course of action. In a democracy such as ours, a forum should exist for all points of view to be expressed. It may be difficult for an individual to accept society's decision concerning a particular ethical dilemma. A physician may be unalterably opposed to the performance of abortion: It is ethical for this physician to discuss a requested abortion as well as other options with the patient, making his or her views known. If this patient requests the abortion, it is incumbent upon the physician to refer the patient to another clinician whose views correspond more closely to those of the patient. Shannon and DiGiacomo, two ethicists, describe five precepts commonly employed by physicians faced with dilemmas in daily practice (Shannon, 1979):

1. The principle of sanctity of life
2. The principle of double effect
3. The principle of totality
4. The principle of justice
5. The principles of religion

The Principle of Sanctity of Life

Ethical, religious, and social precepts of modern western and eastern civilizations recognize the value or sanctity of individual human life. The importance of the individual—his or her right to exist without inappropriate social, economic, medical, or political interference—is one of the primary tenets of our democracy. Both the oath of Hippocrates and the oath of Maimonides, commonly cited credos of the medical profession, include the concept of the sanctity of life.

The Principle of Double Effect

The ethical principle of double effect is employed in situations where a specific clinical decision or intervention can produce two effects: one desirable and hence good, and one undesirable and hence bad. An example of this dilemma is the individual with a malignancy who is being considered for chemotherapy. The goal and expected result of chemotherapy is amelioration of the patient's condition with subsequent prolonged survival (good). However, chemotherapy is associated with numerous painful and even potentially fatal side effects (bad). Ethicists and physicians agree that such an action, with combined good and bad aspects, can be acceptable (1) if the benefit to be gained outweighs the potential harm done, (2) if there is no alternative, less harmful strategy that can be employed, (3) if the action taken does not aim only at immediate minor benefit with definite long-term harm to follow, and (4) if the patient elects to take this action after being informed of the benefits and the risks.

Another category of the principle of double effect is the concept of ordinary versus extraordinary therapeutic interventions. It goes without saying that physicians strive to treat patients to the best of their abilities. However, what happens when routine therapy is ineffective? Should the physician offer the patient experimental or unproved therapies? Should the physician ever give up and offer the patient treatment that only relieves pain and suffering, or should he or she continue to employ one therapeutic strategy after another in an effort to reverse even the most terminal illness? Physicians differ in their tolerance of unremitting therapeutic attempts; some cease such efforts sooner than others. The physician and the patient, working in therapeutic alliance, must decide on that point in a critically ill patient's course when further therapeutic effort only leads to greater suffering without hope of improved quality of life or survival.

The Principle of Totality

This ethical concept states that a part exists for the sake of the whole. Thus, it is ethically justified for the patient to undergo removal of a diseased kidney in order to save his or her life. However, selling of a healthy kidney for profit would seem to be an ethical problem. Risking one's life for economic gain creates a clear ethical dilemma for both patient and physician.

The Principle of Justice

Justice requires that each individual patient be given considerate and equal care. Ideally, the physician's dedication to his or her patient should be without regard to economic status, race, religion, gender, or political viewpoint. Of course, not all patients with the same illness receive identical care across the United States. However, the individual physician should strive to deliver concerned, dedicated care to all patients regardless of their station in life or their racial or religious background. This principle is strained by self-destructive patients such as chronic alcoholics and drug addicts. The physician must recognize his or her own disapproval of these patients as well as the fact that the self-destructive tendency is an illness. It is not expected that the physician psychologically care for every patient. However, it is incumbent upon the physician to attempt to provide good medical care for every patient. Good medical care includes some empathy, some kindness, and of course, conscientiousness.

The Principles of Religion

As noted earlier, the religions of the world recognize the sanctity of life. Moreover, all religions emphasize justice, honesty, and kindness and empathy towards one's fellow men and women. Some religious teachings conflict with others concerning the performance of certain medical procedures (e.g., abortion). In our opinion, there is no right or wrong answer to such religious disagreements. Each physician should consider his or her own beliefs and those of the patient in approaching controversial areas in the clinical arena. Open and frank discussions between physician and patient are the only route to resolution of such problems:

A pregnant 25-year-old sees her gynecologist and requests a therapeutic abortion. The gynecologist opposes abortion on ethical and religious grounds. In the ensuing discussion, the gynecologist openly discusses her opposition to abortion on moral grounds and freely offers to refer the patient *without* recrimination to another gynecologist for the abortion procedure. The patient accepts and may well return to her regular gynecologist for gynecologic follow-up.

Confidentiality

Medical codes of ethics (e.g., the Hippocratic oath) contain statements referring to patient confidentiality. Details of the patient's illness should be kept confidential: Only the physician and the patient need know about them. Of course, parents of a pediatric patient have a right to know the details of their child's illness. Similarly, immediate family members may be informed concerning a patient's illness *if the patient agrees* to such disclosure. Ethical dilemmas arise when family members telephone the physician and request information about a patient's illness. Since the details of the illness are confidential between the patient and the physician, such telephone calls may be difficult for the physician. We propose the following solution: Family members are only given general answers such as "She is in stable (or serious) condition." or "He is undergoing tests, the results of which are not back yet. Please call again after I have discussed the matter fully with the patient." The physician then asks the patient if it is alright to discuss details of the illness with family members. Often discussions between the physician and the patient can take place in the presence of family members so that no secrets are kept by one member of the family from other family members.

Similar physician requests for permission to discuss details of an illness with family members are often appropriate when the patient is an adolescent. Teenagers sometimes guard their privacy and view parental involvement in their medical care (particularly if it deals with sexual matters) with great concern. Again, only a frank discussion between the physician and the patient can resolve such a dilemma.

Research

The medical advances of the last 100 years could not have occurred without extensive animal and human experimentation. However, such experiments involve risk and discomfort for humans and discomfort as well as death for experimental animals. How can an ethically sensitive physician accept such negative effects, even in the search for therapies that lead to reduced suffering and prolonged life? Two ethical principles are involved in decisions concerning experimental medicine: the principle of double effect and the concept of informed consent. The principle of double effect (see p. 160) allows for interventions that lead to both good and bad outcomes as long as good features outweigh negative ones. Thus, it may be ethically acceptable for a patient to volunteer for an experiment that involves some discomfort but that may lead to an improved form of therapy for this patient or others with the same illness. Similarly, investigators using animals in research must be convinced of the importance and the validity of their experimental protocol, and protocols must endeavor to cause the experimental animal as little discomfort as possible.

The concept of informed consent must be involved in all human experiments. It is a legal requirement that each subject of an investigation be informed in understandable terms concerning all aspects of the research protocol, including the expected risks and benefits as well as the potential to withdraw from the experiment at any time.

A young physician approaches a patient with an acute myocardial infarction to discuss the patient's participation in an experimental protocol that involves attempts to dissolve the patient's coronary thrombosis with intravenous streptokinase. The patient is clearly distraught as a result of fear and discomfort. The physician is uncomfortable because she feels that true *informed* consent is difficult to obtain in this setting. The ethical dilemma is resolved by explaining the risks and benefits of the planned protocol to both the patient and his family who have accompanied him. The patient and his family accept the experimental therapy.

All human experimental protocols in the United States are examined by a research board to ensure that the proposed experimental protocol is ethical and that informed consent will be obtained.

Of course, no administrative committee can completely protect a patient's rights. In the final analysis, such protection must rest in the ethical behavior of the physician experimenter.

Literature and Medicine: The Human Perspective*

Helle Mathiasen

It is impossible for medical students or young physicians to experience many ethical dilemmas in their short careers. Consequently, they can only prepare themselves for such issues through reading and discussion. Many works of art and literature present poignant insights into the ethical and personal problems confronting physicians. The question of this era is whether human beings will control the enormous forces unleashed by the scientific and technologic advances of the last 30 years, or whether these forces will result in the annihilation of the human race. The challenge increases in magnitude as scientific and technologic advances continue to accelerate. Decisions made by individuals in our society during the next two decades will determine whether human beings will control science and technology, or whether, in fact, the avalanche of scientific and technologic knowledge will lead to the destruction of life on earth as we know it.

In no other area of science are traditional humanistic concerns expressed more clearly or frequently than in medicine. Indeed, one can make a strong case for the metaphor depicting medicine as the shoreline where the sea of science meets the land mass of the humanities. The implications are evident: If future generations are to learn to control the forces of science and technology, widespread discussion, education, and evaluation of moral, ethical, social, and psychologic aspects of science must be undertaken by medical personnel as well as by society at large.

Certain works of literature, especially those written by physicians or patients, offer insights into the humanistic side of medicine (i.e., that part of the profession that deals not with science but with human beings, the physicians and their patients). Chekhov

*The material used in this essay stems from a collaborative teaching effort between Joseph S. Alpert, M.D., and Helle Mathiasen, Ph.D., in the Honors Program at Boston College, Boston, Massachusetts.

(1860–1904), a man of sensitivity and devotion to his profession as a physician, shows the impossibility of medical progress, even of effective medical care, in an environment of pettiness, corruption, and ignorance, in his novella *Ward Number Six.* Solzhenitsyn (1918–   ), in his novel *Cancer Ward,* gives a fictionalized account of his own experience as a patient in a cancer hospital in the U.S.S.R., dramatizing the terror and helplessness felt by the patient with a corrosive disease. In a lighter vein, the comedy *Knock* by Jules Romains (1885–1972) portrays the country doctor as confidence man, using the gullibility of his community to build himself a position of money and power.

Both medicine and literature are humanistic arts. They resemble each other in their objects, effects, and aims. The object of medicine is humankind. In the laboratory, the medical scientist uses the abstract symbols of science to pinpoint the laws governing the human organism. By the patient's bedside, the practicing physician translates those abstract symbols to fit the case of human need before him or her. In their own ways, workers in medicine seek to expand the limits of our knowledge about ourselves and to use that knowledge for the relief of suffering and the promotion of well-being. Literature, too, has humanity for its object of study. The poet, using words as tools, demonstrates and communicates his or her awareness of the complexity of life. Like the physician, the poet tries first to grasp, then to control, the reality of the human predicament. The effect of medicine when applied is to confer pleasure by relieving pain. The poet, too, gives pleasure to those enjoying his or her art. Finally, the aim of both disciplines is victory, however temporary, over death, the destroyer of life. Both the poet and the physician expend extraordinary amounts of time and energy to ward off death and thus achieve immortality.

In a letter to G. I. Rossolimo dated October 1899, Chekhov, himself a physician and a poet, confirms the relationship between medicine and literature in his own life:

"I have no doubt that the study of medicine has had an important influence on my literary work; it has considerably enlarged the sphere of my observation, has enriched me with a knowledge the true value of which for me as a writer can only be understood by one who is himself a doctor."

Illness is an event that occurs in everyone's life. In most cases, illness becomes a crisis for the patient; furthermore, this crisis and its consequences permanently alter the sufferer and his or her surrounding relationships. A number of questions and issues relating to the study of medicine (e.g., illness, death, and the patient experience) are portrayed in various works of literature: How do patients experience illness? What changes occur in one's self-image due to illness? How does the patient cope with paternalism on the part of the medical profession and with feelings of powerlessness and dependence? What is the distinction between pain and suffering? How do physicians and patients relate on a human level? Should the doctor tell the truth to a dying patient? What are the effects of a variety of medical ethics within the profession (e.g., the pros and cons of loyalty within the medical profession)? What happens when physicians disagree about diagnosis or treatment? What is the definition of a "good" or an "evil" doctor? To what extent should a physician profit from the misfortune of his or her fellow creatures? What effect do societal ethics have on the profession? What is the physician's moral obligation to society and to individual patients?

Finally, diseases have inspired literary works and altered history. Bubonic plague, above all other diseases known to us, has captured the imagination of writers, from Boccaccio (1313–1375) to Camus (1913–1960). Plague epidemics have changed the course of history. In addition, leprosy, syphilis, tuberculosis, typhoid, and typhus have played important roles in art and history.

These issues and many others are raised in a variety of literary works. Life-long reading of nonmedical literature helps to preserve and even intensify a physician's sensitivity to human and ethical issues.

Suggested Reading

DISEASE AS METAPHOR
Camus, A. *The Plague*.
Greene, G. *A Burnt-Out Case*.
Ibsen, H. *Ghosts*.
Mann, T. *The Magic Mountain*.
Poe, E. A. "The Mask of the Red Death."
Solzhenitsyn, A. *Cancer Ward*.

PHYSICIAN PORTRAITS
Cronin, A. J. *The Citadel*.

Hawthorne, N. "Rappacini's Daughter."
Lewis, S. *Arrowsmith.*
Molière. *A Doctor in Spite of Himself* and *The Imaginary Invalid.*
Romains, J. *Knock.*
Stevenson, R. L. *Dr. Jekyll and Mr. Hyde.*

THE EXPERIENCE OF DYING
Tolstoy, L. *The Death of Ivan Ilyich.*

THE EXPERIENCE
OF MENTAL ILLNESS
Kesey, K. *One Flew Over the Cuckoo's Nest.*
Perkins-Gilman, C. *The Yellow Wallpaper.*
Plath, S. *The Bell Jar.*

THE PHYSICIAN AS PATIENT
Lear, M. W. *Heartsounds.* New York: Simon & Schuster, 1980.

THE PHYSICIAN
AS LITERARY ARTIST
Chekhov, A. "The Butterfly," "Ward Number Six," "A Dreary
   Story," "Doctor Startsev," "The Doctor," and "Typhus."
Williams, W. C. *The Autobiography of William Carlos Williams*
   and poems.

BIOETHICS
Brody, H. *Ethical Decisions in Medicine.* Boston: Little, Brown,
   1981.
Papper, S. *Doing Right—Everyday Medical Ethics.* Boston: Little,
   Brown, 1983.
Shannon, T. A., and DiGiacomo, J. J. *An Introduction to Bioethics.*
   New York: Paulist, 1979.

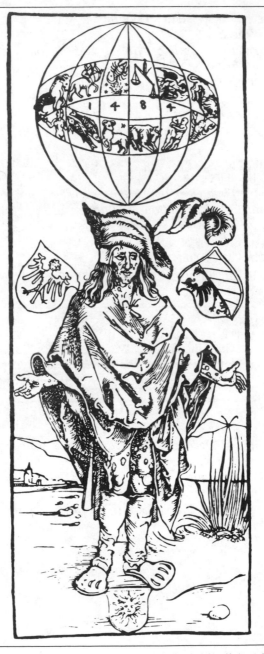

"The Syphilitic." *(A 1484 woodcut by Albrecht Dürer, 1471–1528.)*

20. Bad News

Imparting bad news to a patient is something a physician must be prepared to do from the first to the last day she or he practices medicine. At no other time is the patient in greater need of the physician's empathy and interpersonal skills. At no other time does the physician have a better opportunity to undergo personal growth during a professional task. No matter how many times a physician goes through the experience, the next time is always different—not because there are so many diseases, but because each patient is unique. No matter how well the physician handles the situation, it is never pleasant, but when handled well, it encompasses a physician's most basic mission: to lessen suffering.

Kubler-Ross has outlined a series of stages through which most patients pass after learning of a fatal illness. These stages are shock and denial, anger, bargaining, depression, and acceptance. The physician, especially if she or he has a close relationship with the patient or is of similar age or life circumstances, may also go through some of these stages.

A 25-year-old woman comes to you complaining of easy fatigability and shortness of breath on climbing stairs. She gave birth to her first child one month ago. You suspect that her symptoms reflect fatigue from caring for the baby or even some postpartum depression. However, an examination reveals a heart rate of 120 per minute with a third heart-sound gallop. You become a little anxious, wonder if you are listening correctly, and listen again. Could she be really ill? (Shock and denial) You obtain ventricular function studies, which reveal an ejection fraction of 21 percent. You now know she has a postpartum cardiomyopathy. Damn! (Anger) Your thoughts race. Maybe she will be in the 50 percent of patients who recover. Maybe vigorous treatment with digoxin and unloading agents will give her a better than 50-percent chance. Maybe a biopsy will show inflammation, and steroids or immunosuppressants will help. (Bargaining)

The physician's quick journey past some of the stages through which the patient will go is helpful. It is an empathetic (*em:* in, *pathic:* feeling) process. It heightens your concern and understanding of the patient's feelings. It causes you to search not only for medical solutions but also for ways of dealing with the patient honestly, sensitively, and supportively. The patient will sense this, and it will help his or her confidence and comfort.

The next step is the process of formulating and imparting the bad news to the patient. There are some guidelines for giving bad news.

First, remember that assimilating bad news is a process that takes time. It helps to *give bad news stepwise*. At the first visit of our young patient, one could have laid the groundwork by saying that although one was not entirely sure, a possible reason for the shortness of breath may be a weakening of the heart muscle, something that happens occasionally during or after pregnancy. If asked whether that was serious, one could have answered honestly, while trying not to frighten the patient, "Some people recover quickly while others have more difficulty. I think the best thing to do is to obtain some further tests."

After the confirmatory laboratory information has returned, one must plan a more definitive discussion. Several principles are important here. First is to *take ample time*. Nothing is more frustrating and depressing for the patient than a discussion about serious findings without adequate time to ask questions, voice fears, make plans. If at all possible, *hold the discussion in a private, comfortable place*. This helps the patient vent his or her emotions. If the patient desires it, *allow close family members to be present*. These family members represent support. They may also clarify later for the patient what went on during the discussion. Patients often tune out after the first shock and are not sure what went on. *Think through the presentation ahead of time* so that you are comfortable with it. *Speak simply*, and when possible, *do not use words that have overly negative connotations to the layperson* (i.e., cancer, heart failure). Terms such as "growth" or "weakened heart" will convey the information without the overtones. *Do not say things that will destroy hope*. When the possibility of a benign process or a favorable outcome exists, emphasize it. *Have a treatment plan ready, and state it* along with the bad news. It is very reassuring for the patient to know that there is something that can and will be done; ending on a treatment note suggests hope, not hopelessness. *Assure the patient of your continuing support*. There is a great fear of desertion among patients with serious illness. *Give the patient time and leeway to respond*. It is important that you know how the patient is handling the information and what his or her fears are. *Determine how the diagnosis will affect the patient's life* (i.e., family situation, job).

Not all of these points can be illustrated, but a discussion with our 24-year-old patient might go something like this:

The physician takes the patient into a quiet and comfortable room and asks his office staff not to interrupt him. The visit begins with a warm "How are you feeling?" or "How are you managing with the new baby?" Then it is important to *listen*. There may be questions, fears, that are uppermost in the patient's mind. The patient may also tell the physician directly or indirectly how much she wants to know, or in what time frame. Suppose the patient asks, "What did my tests show?" The physician may respond, "The tests have shown that you do have a weakening of the heart muscle [the bad news]. I am therefore going to begin you on digoxin, a medicine to strengthen your heart [doing something about the problem]. I plan to follow you closely. Together we will work on making you feel better [I will stand by you]." At this point, one might pause and wait for reactions and questions. Before closing, one might ask, "Do you have some help at home with your baby [inquiry about effects of the diagnosis on the patient]?"

Giving bad news is never pleasant for a physician. It goes without saying that receiving the news is even more unpleasant for the patient. Historically, this has caused physicians to withhold or modify the truth at times. In her incisive analysis of this response, Sissela Bok has identified three arguments used by physicians to support this kind of censorship (Bok, 1979): (1) It is impossible to tell the whole truth because we do not know the whole truth. (2) Patients do not really want to hear bad news. (3) Bad news may be harmful, and our most basic philosophic tenet is *Primum non nocere*. Bok goes on to counter each of these arguments very effectively: (1) There is a difference between truth and truthfulness. We may not know everything about a given medical condition, but we certainly can share what we know (i.e., we can be truthful). Anything less is not only contrary to our own moral standards but curtails the patient's right to participate in decisions bearing on his or her illness. (2) Although there is some general feeling that patients do not want to know bad news, actual studies show that 75 to 90 percent of patients who have been asked want the truth. It is too often the physician who does not want to tell and not the patient who does not want to know. The following excerpt from Tolstoy's *The Death of Ivan Ilyich* says it well:

"Ivan Ilyich suffered most of all from the lie, the lie which, for some reason, everyone accepted: that he was not dying but was simply ill, and that if he stayed calm and underwent treatment he could expect good results. Yet he knew that regardless of what was done, all he could expect was more agonizing suffering and death. And he was tortured by this lie, tortured by the fact that they refused to acknowledge what he and everyone else knew, that they wanted to lie about his horrible condition and to force him to become a party to that lie. This lie, a lie perpetrated on the eve of his death, a lie that was bound to degrade the awesome, solemn act of his dying to the level of their social calls, their draperies, the sturgeon they ate for dinner, was an excruciating torture for Ivan Ilyich. And, oddly enough, many times when they were going through their acts with him he came within a hairbreadth of shouting, 'Stop your lying! You and I know that I'm dying, so at least stop lying!' But he never had the courage to do it."

(3) Although bad news can be upsetting, the atmosphere of secrecy or deception is usually worse. Patients tend to deal better with the known than the unknown. They are more compliant, more courageous. It is clear that in order to avoid harming the patient, the timing and the wording as well as the follow-through (see p. 170) are key.

The ability to deal with and communicate bad news is not usually innate. It should be studied, practiced, and critiqued no less than the more technical skills. If anything, it is more difficult than some of the technical tasks, since it requires not only cognitive but also interpersonal expertise. The delivery of bad news marks the beginning of a difficult chapter in a patient's life. The way in which a physician handles it may make an immeasurable difference to the patient. Surely this is a worthy challenge for any physician.

Suggested Reading

Bok, S. *Lying-Moral Choice in Public and Private Life.* New York: Vintage, 1979. Pp. 232–255.

Cassem, N. H. The Dying Patient. *Massachusetts General Hospital Handbook of General Hospital Psychiatry.* St. Louis: Mosby, 1978. Pp. 300–318.

Kübler-Ross, E. *On Death and Dying.* New York: Macmillan, 1969.

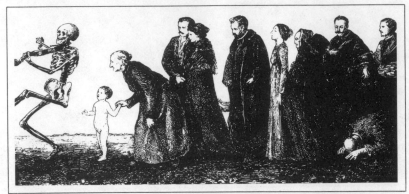

"The Dance of Death." The theme of this drawing, respice finem *(remember your death), has been popular since the Middle Ages. (By Joseph Winkel, nineteenth century.)*

21. Resuscitation and Do Not Resuscitate Orders

When a person dies in the hospital, the initial witness does not always know whether death came as an unexpected, unwanted accident or a welcome release from suffering. Rules dictate that the first person on the scene call a *code*, an emergency call for a designated team to carry out cardiopulmonary resuscitation (CPR). This sequence can be avoided only if a *do not resuscitate* order (DNR) has been written in the chart at some prior time, and the front of the chart has been labeled with the letters DNR.

Do not resuscitate orders have been the subject of much thought and controversy. When is it appropriate to write such orders? What is the effect of the orders on the patient's general care? Absolute answers to these questions are impossible. However, there are some general principles involved in making these decisions. Some examples serve to illustrate both the principles and problems.

A 58-year-old man is admitted to the hospital with pneumonia. Two months ago, he underwent partial colectomy and partial hepatectomy for carcinoma of the colon metastatic to the liver. Two weeks ago, after a full and honest discussion, he accepted his physician's recommendation that he undergo chemotherapy and began his treatments. He understands the seriousness of his illness, but clings to his optimism. His attitude is positive, yet he continuously seeks support from his physician. The house officer who admits him for pneumonia feels that he looks very ill and asks the attending physician about his code status.

The most basic principle when considering *code status* is that the patient's wishes are paramount. The most difficult problem encountered by the physician in this situation is whether, when, and how to ask the patient directly. Some strict advocates of patient autonomy would advise the attending physician always to ask the patient directly about CPR. They would emphasize introducing this subject as early in a serious illness as possible. They would argue that anything less robs the patient of a fundamental right of self-determination. We do not completely agree. Although a patient-initiated request for or against CPR should always be honored, a physician-initiated discussion is not always appropriate nor does it always elicit the patient's real wishes. The physician must judge whether such questioning will be helpful or harmful and whether the outcome reflects the patient's real feelings. *Timing is critical on both counts.* In some instances, general discussions of the illness offer a rather easy opening for discussion of CPR. In other situations, the patient is fragile, and reassurance within the bounds of honesty seems wiser. Not all patients will choose strict autonomy. Not all patients want to hear about all potential complications and the different possible responses to them. Although the principle of patient autonomy is clearly important, it must be coupled with sensitivity and clinical judgment. Timing and the physician's approach temper the accuracy and the effect of a *no code* discussion.

The patient in the first example appears to be *competent, informed,* and *critically,* but at this juncture *not terminally, ill.* He has indirectly signaled *his wish* to live by accepting chemotherapy. He has also signaled his physician in many ways that emotionally he is not ready for a discussion of resuscitation. We feel that he should be given a full code and not be queried directly at this time about his desires with respect to resuscitation.

Let us suppose that the patient goes on to have a cardiopulmonary arrest and survives resuscitation. At that point in time, the patient may very well bring up the subject of whether ever to repeat CPR. Alternatively, his physician, in discussing the events with him retrospectively, may find it very easy to raise the question of a repeat code with much less chance of introducing unwanted fears. These scenarios demonstrate how principles must be coupled with sensitivity and clinical judgment.

The same 58-year-old man has recovered from his pneumonia without CPR. He is improved after his chemotherapy. He returns to work for about 8 months and then develops progressive weakness and increasing abdominal pain. X-ray examinations show widespread metastases. The patient has asked about the x rays and has been told the truth kindly. He has been offered another course of chemotherapy but has refused. He finally asks to be hospitalized in order not to burden his family. He specifically requests not to be kept alive by artificial means. He also asks that he be kept as free of pain as possible since he enjoys seeing his family when he is not preoccupied with pain. Once again, the house officer asks the physician about the patient's code status.

In this situation, discussion of CPR as one of the possibilities seems much less apt to harm the patient's spirits. Let us say that such a discussion occurs and the patient asks not to be resuscitated. Since the patient is *competent,* well informed, and has expressed *his wish* not to be resuscitated, the physician should write a note in the chart documenting the discussion and should write—*not telephone*—the DNR order into the chart.

If the patient had been admitted obtunded or comatose before expressing his feelings about further heroic efforts, the physician would have had to discuss resuscitation with a family member, either someone previously delegated by the patient, or more often, a person chosen by the family at the time. The physician should assure her- or himself that this person is competent, well informed about diagnosis and prognosis, and either the closest relative or the true spokesperson for the closest relative. Sometimes this family member will ask the physician's advice or ask the physician to make the decision. The physician should accept this responsibility and carry it out in what she or he feels to be the patient's best interest. The question of possible legal problems at a later time may enter the physician's mind. If this procedure is followed, such problems are unlikely. However, physicians constantly work in a setting where future legal concerns must be balanced against humanistic care. A distinguished panel including physicians and lawyers has written, "Treatment of a dying patient always takes place in the context of changing social policy, but in spite of legal uncertainties appropriate and compassionate care should have priority over undue fears of criminal or civil liability" (Wanzer, 1984).

Let us suppose that a no code order has been written on the chart of our 58-year-old patient. What is the effect of this order on the care of the patient? No code orders can present emotional problems for physicians. They may convey the feeling that there is nothing active to do for the patient. They may imply that there is no teaching value to the patient. The simple classification of *code* or *no code* status contributes significantly to the problem. It is clearly inadequate. Wanzer et al. have identified several stages in the care of terminally ill patients (Wanzer, 1984):

1. Emergency resuscitation: a full code
2. Intensive care and advanced life support: such things as a respirator but not CPR
3. General medical care, including antibiotics, drugs, surgery, cancer chemotherapy, artificial hydration, and nutrition
4. General nursing care and efforts to make the patient comfortable including pain relief, hydration, and nutrition as dictated by the patient's thirst and hunger

Physicians should seriously consider classifying patients into these categories rather than into code and no code. Our 58-year-old patient falls into category 4, general nursing care and efforts to make the patient comfortable. Good supportive care in this situation means an order to offer pain medication, in ample dosages for pain relief, without undue worry about overdose, and at intervals shorter than those in which severe pain develops. Certainly one should not worry about drug addiction in terminal patients. Good supportive care also means a willingness to listen to the patient, taking time that in other patients might be spent on laboratory reports or diagnostic and therapeutic plans and giving that time to the physician-patient relationship in its purest form. The physician should remember that it is not the fear of dying but the fear of desertion that weighs most heavily on the terminally ill. Moreover, it is important to bear in mind that DNR means "do not resuscitate," *not* "do nothing right."

A totally neglected aspect of the care of terminally ill patients is the effect of impending death on other patients. When the patient is close to death, it may be a kindness to mention the situation to the person in the next bed. It is certainly helpful for that person to know that the serious condition of the patient is known and accepted by physicians and family. An example serves to illustrate this problem:

A 75-year-old man with end-stage renal disease and congestive heart failure is in the same room with a 35-year-old man who is recovering from some injuries. The older patient has refused dialysis. After he becomes comatose, the situation is discussed with the family, and a no code order is written. The physician says to the young roommate, "I needn't tell you that your roommate is very ill and might pass away." "I know, doc," he says. "I've been watching him, and I'm ready to jump into the bed and give him CPR if necessary!" The physician says, "Please don't do that. He is seriously ill, and everyone accepts the fact that nothing more can be done for him. You would only prolong his or the family's suffering." "I'm so glad you told me that, doc," the roommate says. "You know I'm an EMT [emergency medical technician]."

In summary, we must continue to demonstrate to our patients, their families, and those around them that no matter what level of care they are to receive, they are worthy of our time and effort. Perhaps it might help to remember that most of us will reach their status one day. It is not a question of whether this will happen, but only when, where, and how. For the present, we should constantly remind ourselves that no code is not synonymous with no care.

Suggested Reading

Jackson, D. L., and Youngner, S. Patient autonomy and "death with dignity." Some clinical caveats. *N. Engl. J. Med.* 301:404, 1979.

Wanzer, S. H., Adelstein, S. J., Cranford, R. E., Federman, D. D., Hook, E. D., Moertel, C. G., Safar, P., Stone, A., Taussig, H. B., and Van Eys, J. The physician's responsibility toward hopelessly ill patients. *N. Engl. J. Med.* 310:955, 1984.

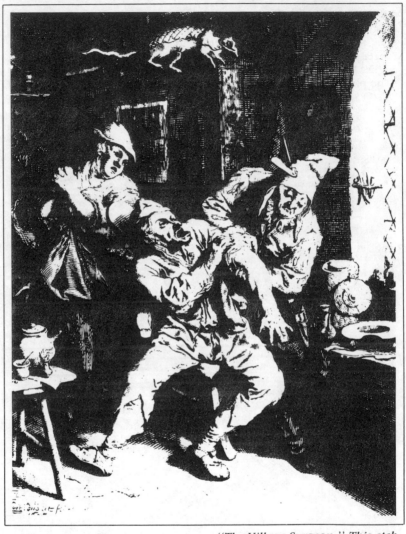

"The Village Surgeon." This etching reveals a rustic village surgeon performing a minor operation on a peasant. Various herbs,
minerals, and animal products
used as medicines can be seen in
the background. (By Cornelius Du-
sart, 1660–1704.)

22. Health Insurance, Disability, Workers' Compensation, and Health Maintenance Organizations

A major factor that has contributed to the growth of the American biomedical complex during the past 50 years has been health insurance coverage for hospital and physician services. In 1940, less than 10 percent of the American population had health insurance coverage for inpatient care. At the present time, approximately 80 percent of American citizens under age 65 and virtually all citizens over age 65 have health insurance covering both hospital and physician services. A variety of different health insurance plans and coverage schemes exist, ranging from individual private policies covering a single person to extensive group plans covering thousands of individuals.

Blue Cross–Blue Shield and Other Private Health Insurance Plans

Blue Cross–Blue Shield is a nonprofit, nontaxable corporation that sells health insurance throughout the country. Every state has its own Blue Cross–Blue Shield organization. Hospital services are covered by Blue Cross, while physician fees are reimbursed by Blue Shield. In many cases, hospitals and physicians accept the reimbursed amount of money as payment in full. This is called *accepting assignment*. In some states, Blue Cross–Blue Shield–participating physicians must accept assignment. In other states, hospitals and physicians collect a supplemental fee (above the amount reimbursed by health insurance) from the patient. Health insurance is usually part of the fringe-benefit package that workers receive from their employers. The latter usually pay most or all of the health insurance premiums. Industries with large numbers of employees are generally able to negotiate more extensive coverage policies for their employees because the rate of payment is shared among a large number of individuals. A similar financing strategy lies behind health maintenance organizations (HMOs).

Most health insurance plans require that the patient or family unit covered pay a certain fixed amount, the deductible, in each calendar year before coverage takes effect. Deductibles usually range from $50 to $300. There are a very large number of different benefit packages, with private individual policies offering the least extensive coverage and large group plans offering the best benefits. For example, a major medical plan of Blue Cross–Blue Shield covers 80 percent of inpatient and outpatient services, while a comprehensive policy covers 100 percent of inpatient expenses and 100 percent of outpatient services.

Medicare

Medicare is a federal health insurance plan for individuals over 65 years of age and severely disabled patients under 65 years of age. (Disability is discussed on p. 184.) The money for Medicare insurance comes from Social Security funds. Medicare insurance is divided into two parts. Part A is coverage for inpatient services; part B helps pay for physician services, outpatient visits, and other medical items not covered by part A (e.g., a wheelchair or hospital bed to be used at home). Part A also covers treatment in extended care facilities for posthospital convalescence (e.g., rehabilitation) as well as home health services (e.g., physical therapy home visits). The patient pays nothing for part A, which is completely financed by the federal government. Part B is optional and is financed partly by the government (50%) and partly by the individual (50%) through monthly premium payments. Part B is usually administered by Blue Cross–Blue Shield. The effect of deductibles, limitations on coverage, and service exclusions (i.e., routine dental and visual care) means that individuals over age 65 end up paying for approximately half of their health care expenditures. Under part B, patients are reimbursed for 80 percent of most outpatient services such as office visits, laboratory tests, and x rays. Some supplemental plans to Medicare reimburse 80 percent of the cost of prescription drugs after a deductible.

Medicaid

The Medicaid program is completely separate from Medicare. Medicaid is part of the welfare system and was developed to assist indigent patients. Funding from Medicaid is 50 to 80 percent federal government and 20 to 50 percent state government depending on the individual state's economy. Some states have very meager welfare programs and obtain very little federal Medicaid funding. There is, therefore, great variability from state to state in the adequacy of the Medicaid program. Medicaid reimbursement rates are usually quite low, a fact that has led to hostility towards the program from health care providers. Blue Cross–Blue Shield generally reimburses physicians in the range of 67 cents for each dollar billed (depending on community, physician, and in- or outpatient service). For example, these insurers would pay a physician approximately $65 for a bill of $100. Medicaid, however, only reimburses in the range of 10 to 20 cents for each dollar billed. Thus, the physician who submits a bill for $100 is only paid approximately $15 by Medicaid. Participating providers (physicians and hospitals) are not allowed to seek supplemental payment from Medicaid patients.

Champus

Champus is an abbreviation for Civilian Health and Medical Program of the Uniformed Services. It is a health insurance program that covers dependents of active military personnel and retired military personnel and their families. Inpatient and outpatient services are covered, although the patient must shoulder approximately 20 percent of the health care bill. Retired military personnel must have served for 20 years in order to be eligible for Champus benefits for themselves and their families. Such retirees are also eligible to receive care from military hospitals and clinics and from Veterans Administration hospitals.

Veterans Administration Hospitals

Veterans of military service who have served under 20 years of active service are not eligible for military hospital care or Champus coverage. These individuals are, however, eligible to receive care from Veterans Administration (VA) hospitals and clinics if their income is less than a specific amount. Individuals with military service–related disability are eligible for care at VA facilities regardless of income. All care in VA facilities is free since all personnel (including physicians) are paid by the federal government. Inpatient VA facilities are more common than outpatient programs; however, outpatient programs also offer physician care and medication without cost to recipients.

Disability

Patients who are totally and permanently disabled are eligible to receive Medicare health insurance benefits even though they have not reached age 65. In addition, patients with chronic renal failure have their dialysis and other medical expenses covered under the disability section of Medicare. Totally and permanently disabled individuals must be disabled for 1 year before they can receive Medicare health benefits and Social Security living expenses. Physicians are often called upon to offer an opinion as to whether an individual is truly "permanently and totally" disabled. This can lead to a very difficult decision for the physician since the patient is often urging the doctor to declare him or her disabled. Many guidelines have been published to aid physicians in this decision. However, in the final analysis, the physician must employ his or her knowledge of the patient, the patient's illness, and the demands of the patient's job in rendering a final recommendation for or against the disability category. The situation is complicated by varying disability requirements, depending on the nature of the patient's disability insurance. Thus, certain policies demand that the patient be disabled for *any and all* employment before payment is made. Other policies (more expensive) only require the patient to be disabled with respect to his current job. Middle-aged patients with moderate disability may be caught in the horns of an even nastier dilemma: They cannot perform their current job; they are not disabled sufficiently to qualify for their disability insurance, which states "disabled for any and all employment"; and finally they are too old to be able to find alternative employment. Consequently, some of the most unpleasant psychologic situations of medical practice occur in the setting of disability applications.

Workers' Compensation

Each state has its own workers' compensation legislation, which requires employers of more than a specific number of employees to carry medical and living expense disability insurance for employees whose injuries or illnesses are the result of their employment. Workers' compensation health insurance covers both in- and outpatient services and medications. In the case of job-related injuries, there is usually little debate as to whether the worker is eligible for coverage under workers' compensation insurance. However, illnesses that begin at work are often said by the patient to be job-related even though the physician may be skeptical. This is another example of a situation that may lead to disagreement between physician and patient. As in the case of disability assessment, the patient often wishes the physician to make a specific declaration: The patient is totally and permanently disabled, or the patient's illness is job-related. The physician, on the other hand, may feel that the patient is not disabled or the illness is unrelated to the patient's employment. An example of the type of unpleasant situation that can arise follows:

A 50-year-old woman suffers a myocardial infarction. She has multiple risk factors for coronary artery disease: heavy cigarette smoking for 25 years, moderate hypertension, a serum cholesterol of 325 mg per dl, and a family history of myocardial infarction in women younger than 50 years of age. The patient's chest pain that led to hospitalization for myocardial infarction developed while she was at work. During her convalescence, the patient informs her physician that she is "convinced that my heart attack was caused by stress on my job." The patient applies for workers' compensation benefits and is denied them because her physician, who understands the role of the patient's multiple, long-standing risk factors, refuses to state that the patient's myocardial infarction is the result of job-related stress. The patient-physician relationship is severely strained.

There is no simple solution to such dilemmas. The physician must examine each case of this nature with care and understanding. If the physician feels that the patient is probably not disabled or the illness or injury is probably not job-related, he or she should state this clearly to the patient before a misunderstanding can develop.

Health Maintenance Organizations

Health maintenance organizations, or prepaid group practice plans, are independent, often free-standing institutions that offer comprehensive health care benefits including in- and outpatient services. The patient joins an HMO instead of obtaining health care insurance such as Blue Cross–Blue Shield. The individual (and usually the employer) pay a yearly premium to the HMO, which then provides the patient with inpatient and outpatient health care for that year. Often a small fee ($2–3) is charged for each visit to the HMO pharmacy or dentist. If specialty consultations are needed, the patient is referred to the required specialist within the HMO. The HMO itself may operate an outpatient clinic, a hospital, and even a rehabilitation facility, or it may contract for hospital services from private institutions in the community it serves.

Health maintenance organizations usually offer far more comprehensive benefits than the usual health insurance programs. The yearly premium for the HMO is often less expensive. Health maintenance organization coverage often includes medications and routine eye and dental care.

A drawback to HMO care is that the subscriber has no choice or very limited choice of physician and hospital. A recently formed alternative to the HMO is the individual practice association (IPA), or preferred provider organization (PPO). This entity exploits the weakness of HMOs (i.e., limited choice). An IPA or PPO consists of a large group of physicians as well as hospitals in an area who band together and contract with the IPA to offer services to patients at a fixed rate. This alternative form of prepaid health insurance incorporates a broad range of physicians who are already in practice and accessible to the enrolled population. Physicians are reimbursed at predetermined fee-for-service rates by the IPA (PPO) administration. The IPAs (PPOs) have developed rapidly in communities where HMOs are making inroads into traditional physician practices. The physicians in the area use the IPA as a defense against patient recruitment by the HMO.

Suggested Reading

Kramer, D. C. *Medical Practice Management.* Boston: Little, Brown, 1982. Pp. 109–116.

Social Security Regulations: Rules for Determining Disability and Blindness. U. S. Department of Health and Human Services. SSA publication No. 64-014, 1981.

Williams, S. J., and Torrens, P. R. *Introduction to Health Services.* New York: 1980. Pp. 17–28, 303–316.

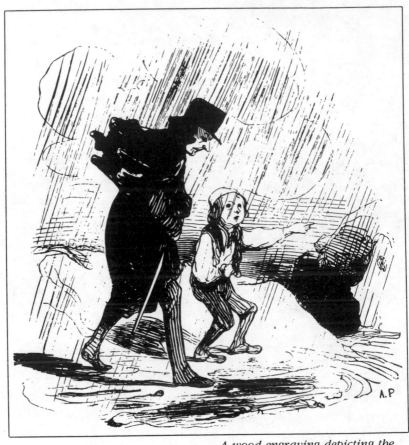

A wood engraving depicting the quiet devotion of a country doctor, called out in a storm to pay a house call. (Engraving after Honoré Daumier, 1808–1879. From Fabre's Nemesis Medicale. *Paris, 1840.)*

23. Physician Images

Physician images have undergone striking alterations over the centuries from the select priesthood of the Hippocratic era (approximately 500 B.C.), through the Latin-speaking and ineffectual pedant of Molière, to the kindly but stern physician of Norman Rockwell's paintings. During the past 2 decades, the image of the physician has shifted again, to that of a scientific, highly technical, and cold individual often with too little time for patients or family.

". . . the doctors . . . were with him for ten minutes a day. They were marginal figures, shadowy and cold. They touched him with instruments— stethoscopes, blood-pressure gadgets. They had condescending airs. They asked him many curt questions and grunted at him. He did not like them. . . . How quickly arrogance had been bred. . . . How early they grew pompous!" (Lear, 1980)

In juxtaposition to this negative image, however, is that of the all-knowing, compassionate, and all too perfect physician portrayed in a variety of popular television programs such as "Marcus Welby," "Trapper John, M.D.," and "Quincy." It is thus not surprising that the American public has ambiguous and conflicting feelings about physicians in general, although surveys have demonstrated that most Americans do have strongly positive feelings about their own physicians.

Literary depictions of physicians have emphasized both negative and positive qualities. Negative characteristics include greed, lechery, self-importance, arrogance, and pedantry. Portrayals of such unpleasant physicians are readily apparent in literary works such as Molière's *The Imaginary Invalid* and *The Doctor in Spite of Himself*, Sinclair Lewis's *Arrowsmith*, A. J. Cronin's *The Citadel*, and Tolstoy's *The Death of Ivan Ilyich*, among others. Positive physician qualities portrayed in literature include compassion, warmth, tireless effort on behalf of the patient, and honesty. Physicians with such positive characteristics can be found in Camus's *The Plague*, A. J. Cronin's *The Citadel*, and Sinclair Lewis's *Arrowsmith*, among others. We encourage physicians to read some of these works alone or in seminar groups. Good literature prompts us to see and think about ourselves.

Each physician possesses the potential to develop into a compassionate, dedicated healer. That is, of course, what motivated most of us to become physicians in the first place. On the other hand, we are also capable of becoming hardened, cruel, and indifferent, given the various pressures and stresses to which we are subject. It is our contention that each physician should periodically reflect and meditate on those positive and desirable qualities that should characterize our profession. We believe that most physicians do just this and that truly evil physicians are rare.

Unfortunately, mass media frequently emphasize the unusual physician who is portrayed as acquisitive, distant, and apt to cover up serious errors in his or her medical practice. Of course, the medical profession is not the only group whose less admirable members receive media attention: Aberrant lawyers, teachers, business executives, and politicians are often played up as well. However, members of these professions are usually not expected to dedicate themselves to the aid and comfort of their fellow humans to the same degree that physicians are. Thus, the evil physician arouses greater public revulsion than the evil lawyer or business executive. In short, Americans expect more of their doctors and are, consequently, more outraged when physicians fall short of the mark. Physicians carry a burden of expected saintly behavior regardless of their actual life situations. Physicians' images of themselves are as complex and many-faceted as the public conception of the profession. Over-worked, often unappreciated for their long hours of effort, and expected to behave with unending patience and self-control, many physicians become disillusioned and exhausted after 10 to 20 years of practice. The discrepancy between what is expected of them and what they can do becomes too much for many middle-aged physicians, who then seek relief by changes in career or personal life.

Is there a solution to the dilemma just described: the incongruity between the public image of the physician and the individual physician's ability to live up to this image? Complete resolution of this problem is probably not possible. Media coverage of medical miracles will continue to raise public expectation of physician performance even for the gravest illness. At the same time, most physicians want to reassure and support their patients. This combination of public expectation and the physician's desire to support and reassure can lead patients to expect unrealistic results from the medical care system. It is important for physicians to describe honestly and fully the prognosis for improvement. However, physicians should avoid the temptation to paint an overly bleak picture for the patient and his or her family. Physicians need to give themselves time to relate to patients and time to reflect on their own lives and behavior. Moreover, physicians should educate and inform their patients so that the latter do not harbor false expectations. Consider the following example:

A young physician feels a flush of pleasure when a basically healthy patient praises him for his wonderful care, which led to rapid resolution of her bronchopneumonia. This sense of elation is rapidly replaced by irritation when the next patient, an elderly man with metastatic carcinoma of the prostate, rebukes the physician for "not doing anything to help me." An unpleasant and hostile confrontation ensues.

In this example, the young physician was elated by his effective therapeutic regimen for the first patient. His sense of pleasure arose from the recognition by the patient of the physician's curative power. This elation rapidly disappeared, however, when the physician was confronted with a patient whom he could not cure, a man with metastatic cancer. The unpleasant scene that followed was the result of two false images of the physician: (1) the first patient's (and the physician's own) false image of physician power, and (2) the second patient's false expectation of physician performance even in the face of mortal illness. A more effective response on the part of the physician would have been to say to the first patient, "Yes, things have gone well with your illness because effective antibiotics were available to destroy the bacteria that were causing your pneumonia. Unfortunately, modern medicine, despite advances, can't cure many illnesses, and it is a pleasure for me to participate in the cure of patients like yourself." To the second patient, the physician should have said, "I know how you feel since, of course, I cannot destroy your tumor. But I may be able to control its spread, and I will certainly do everything I can to minimize your pain. I will stand by you in this difficult time and, working together, we will see you through this." Dialogues like these emphasize the real ability of physician to comfort and occasionally to cure. They aid both patients in understanding what modern medicine can and cannot do. They also remind the physician what he or she can and cannot do. Hopefully, false expectations will gradually fade, and a more realistic view of the medical profession's abilities will prevail.

Suggested Reading

Camus, A. *The Plague.*
Cronin, A. J. *The Citadel.*
Lear, M. W. *Heartsounds.* New York: Simon & Schuster, 1980. Pp. 40–41.
Lewis, S. *Arrowsmith.*
Tolstoy, L. *The Death of Ivan Ilyich.*

Appendixes

A. Medical Oaths and Codes

Oath of Maimonides

Thy eternal providence has appointed me to watch over the life and health of my fellow human beings. May the love for my art actuate me at all times: May neither avarice nor miserliness, nor thirst for glory, or for great reputation engage my mind; for the enemies of truth and philanthropy could easily deceive me and make me forgetful of my lofty aim of doing good to my patients. May I never see in the patient anything but a fellow creature of pain. Grant me strength, time, and opportunity, always to correct what I have acquired, always to extend its domain; for knowledge is immense and the spirit of man can extend infinitely to enrich itself daily with new requirements. Today we can discover our errors of yesterday, and tomorrow we may obtain a new light on what we think ourselves sure of today.

I have been appointed to watch over the life and death of my fellow human beings. Here am I ready for my vocation, and now I turn unto my calling.

Oath of Hippocrates

I swear by Apollo, the Physician, and Aesculapius and health and all-heal and all the Gods and Goddesses that, according to my ability and judgment, I will keep this oath and stipulation:

To reckon him who taught me this art equally dear to me as my parents, to share my substance with him and relieve his necessities if required: to regard his offspring as on the same footing with my own brothers, and to teach them this art if they should wish to learn it, without fee or stipulation, and that by precept, lecture, and every other mode of instruction, I will impart a knowledge of the art to my own sons and to those of my teachers, and to disciples bound by a stipulation and oath, according to the law of medicine, but to none others.

I will follow that method of treatment which, according to my ability and judgment, I consider for the benefit of my patients, and abstain from whatever is deleterious and mischevious. I will give no deadly medicine to anyone if asked, nor suggest any such counsel; furthermore, I will not give to a woman an instrument to produce abortion.

With Purity and with Holiness I will pass my life and practice my art. I will not cut a person who is suffering with a stone, but will leave this to be done by practitioners of this work. Into whatever houses I enter I will go into them for the benefit of the sick and will abstain from every voluntary act of mischief and corruption; and further from the seduction of females or males, bond or free.

Whatever, in connection with my professional practice, or not in connection with it, I may see or hear in the lives of men which ought not to be spoken abroad I will not divulge, as reckoning that all such should be kept secret. While I continue to keep this oath unviolated may it be granted to me to enjoy life and the practice of the art, respected by all men at all times but should I trespass and violate this oath, may the reverse be my lot.

Declaration of Geneva *

At the time of being admitted as a member of the medical profession:
>   I will give to my teachers the respect and gratitude which is their due;
>   I will practice my profession with conscience and dignity;
>   The health of my patient will be my first consideration;
>   I will respect the secrets which are confided in me, even after the patient has died;
>   I will maintain by all the means in my power the honor and the noble traditions of the medical profession;
>   My colleagues will be my brothers;
>   I will not permit considerations of religion, nationality, race, party politics or social standing to intervene between my duty and my patient;
>   I will maintain the utmost respect for human life from the time of conception; even under threat, I will not use my medical knowledge contrary to the laws of humanity;
>   I make these promises solemnly, freely and upon my honor.

Preamble to the American Medical Association Principles of Medical Ethics

The medical profession has long subscribed to a body of ethical statements developed primarily for the benefit of the patient. As a member of this profession, a physician must recognize responsibility not only to patients, but also to society, to other health professionals, and to self. The following principles adopted by the American Medical Association are not laws, but standards of conduct which define the essentials of honorable behavior for the physician.

  I. A physician shall be dedicated to providing competent medical service with compassion and respect for human dignity.
  II. A physician shall deal honestly with patients and colleagues and strive to expose those physicians deficient in character or competence, or who engage in fraud or deception.
  III. A physician shall respect the law and also recognize a responsibility to seek changes in those requirements which are contrary to the best interests of the patient.
  IV. A physician shall respect the rights of patients, of colleagues, and of

*Instituted in 1948 and amended in 1968.

other health professionals, and shall safeguard patient confidences within the constraints of the law.

V. A physician shall continue to study, apply, and advance scientific knowledge; make relevant information available to patients, colleagues, and the public; obtain consultation; and use the talents of other health professionals when indicated.

VI. A physician shall, in the provision of appropriate patient care, except in emergencies, be free to choose whom to serve, with whom to associate, and the environment in which to provide medical services.

VII. A physician shall recognize a responsibility to participate in activities contributing to an improved community.

B. Community Services

Care of the patient does not end when that individual is discharged from the hospital. All physicians expect to follow their patients in an outpatient setting following discharge. Less well known are the myriad services available to patients in the community to which they return. These services are often staffed by volunteers and are frequently funded from municipal, state, federal, or charitable sources. Hence, the cost to the patient is minimal or nonexistent. Knowledge of community resources is the area of expertise of social workers. These health professionals invariably have a wealth of information concerning such resources, and they should be consulted as soon as the physician becomes aware that a potential problem may exist following the patient's discharge from the hospital. This chapter contains brief descriptions of *some* community resources with an example of their usefulness in patient care.

Home Health Agencies

Very few physicians make house calls anymore. This form of medical care delivery is usually seen as inefficient and, therefore, wasteful of medical resources. Although this claim is probably true, much important information about the patient's illness and the best way to manage it can be obtained from an examination of the patient's home environment. Most American cities and towns have at least one organization that specializes in making house calls, thereby furnishing the physician with information about the patient's home situation. Most often staffed by nurses, such organizations as the Visiting Nurses Association (VNA) will make up to several visits per week to patients with ongoing medical problems. Most or all of these services are paid for by various health insurance plans so that the cost to the patient is usually minimal. Visiting nurses keep in close touch with the patient's physician, informing him or her of the patient's status, home environment, and adherence to therapy. Often, such information results in important decisions that can lead to marked improvement in the patient's condition.

A 75-year-old man who has recently lost his wife is admitted to the hospital with an acute inferior myocardial infarction complicated by left ventricular failure. The patient stabilizes on a medical regimen containing four different pharmacologic preparations. At the time of discharge from the hospital, the patient, a fiercely independent individual, insists that he will have no problem caring for himself once he returns home. Five days after hospital discharge, the attending physician receives a call from the visiting nurse who has seen the patient twice. The nurse reports that the patient lives in a large apartment, knows very little about food preparation, and is overwhelmed by the prospect of cooking and housekeeping, although adamantly denying any feelings of insecurity. After a brief discussion, the physician and nurse consult a social worker, who assists them in obtaining supportive services for the patient. Shortly thereafter, a part-time housekeeper and home health aide begin visiting the patient regularly to help with house cleaning, shopping, cooking, and adherence to the prescribed medical program. The patient is thereby enabled to continue living in his apartment.

This type of situation occurs almost daily in older patients. Elderly or handicapped individuals, striving for independence, overestimate their physical endurance or resources at home. Their independent existence is thereby threatened, and they face admission to a chronic care facility such as a nursing home. Most of these individuals prefer to remain in their own apartment or home and can continue to do so with appropriate community support. Many communities have special centers for aged or handicapped individuals. Such centers supply occupational, recreational, and daily living assistance, which varies, of course, from center to center. It is not uncommon, however, for these centers to supply meals, recreational and occupational counseling and therapy, and even assistance in the patient's home. Often, such agencies can assist handicapped individuals in obtaining specialized health care equipment to use in their homes. Many communities also have meals-on-wheels programs that will deliver a warm dinner each day to house-bound patients. Hospital social service departments make it a point to be conversant with such community resources.

Nursing Homes

Patients who are incapable of caring for themselves at home and for whom sufficient family or community resources cannot be found for such home care must be admitted to a nursing home where daily basic needs can be met. For the average American, who has lived his or her life in his or her own home or apartment, the institutional existence of a nursing home is a depressing experience. Consequently, independent home existence should be sought whenever possible for patients following discharge from the hospital.

Specific Organizations
for Handicapped Patients

A number of community organizations offer assistance to patients affected by a particular handicap (e.g., loss of sight or hearing). These organizations can assist patients and their families with a variety of practical or psychologic problems that arise as a result of the handicap. Some of the conditions for which specialized community agencies or organizations exist are presented at the end of this appendix.

Protective Organizations

Most communities have agencies and organizations that support and protect battered women and abused children. Most states have enacted legislation to assist such organizations in the defense of such patients. Social service departments are knowledgeable about such legislation and protective organizations available in a given community.

Alcoholism and Drug Abuse Programs

Alcoholics and drug abusers have a high incidence of serious health problems that are the direct result of their substance abuse. Permanent withdrawal from the offending substance is always a major therapeutic goal in such patients. Organizations such as Alcoholics Anonymous and Narcotics Anonymous seek to engage patients in meetings with others who have successfully maintained abstinence from the addicting substance.

These groups seek to support members in maintaining total abstinence from addicting substances. Members of these organizations will usually see patients in the hospital prior to discharge in order to coordinate the patient's participation in the organization after discharge. These organizations seem to offer the most effective means of maintaining sobriety or permanent withdrawal from addicting substances. However, when this is unsuccessful, special inhospital alcohol or drug centers are available. Patients are usually admitted for several weeks for intensive rehabilitative efforts.

Illnesses for Which Specific Community Organizations Exist*

Allergy
Alzheimer's disease
Amyotrophic lateral sclerosis
Anorexia nervosa
Asthma
Autism
Birth defects
Black lung
Blindness
Cancer
Cardiovascular disease
Cerebral palsy
Diabetes
Dyslexia
Hearing loss
Mental retardation
Multiple sclerosis
Musculoskeletal disabilities (e.g., loss of limb)
Obesity
Parkinson's disease

*See Suggested Reading for references that will supply addresses and phone numbers of specific agencies.

Psychiatric disease
Sickle cell disease
Systemic lupus erythematosus
Tay-Sachs disease

Suggested Reading

Kipps, H. C. *Community Resources Directory.* Detroit: Gale, 1984.
Kruzas, A. T. *Social Service Organizations and Agencies Directory.* Detroit: Gale, 1982.
Saunders Health Care Directory 84–85. Philadelphia: Saunders, 1984.

Index

Index